MAY 0 7 2014

MEDICAL SERVICES
IN THE
FIRST WORLD WAR

Susan Cohen

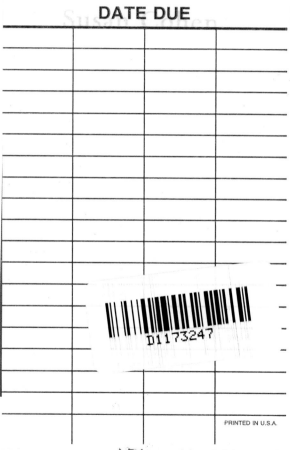

SHIRE PUBLICATIONS

940.475
Cohen

Published in Great Britain in 2014 by Shire Publications
Ltd, PO Box 883, Oxford, OX1 9PL, UK

PO Box 3985, New York, NY 10185-3985, USA

E-mail: shire@shirebooks.co.uk www.shirebooks.co.uk

A CIP catalogue record for this book is available from the
British Library.

Shire Library no. 792. ISBN-13: 978 0 74780 369 9

Susan Cohen has asserted her right under the Copyright,
Designs and Patents Act, 1988, to be identified as the author
of this book.

Designed by Tony Truscott Designs, Sussex, UK and typeset
in Perpetua and Gill Sans.

Cover design and photography by Peter Ashley, with thanks
to an English Heritage Festival of History enactment;
back cover detail from Our Hospital ABC (Peter Ashley's
collection).

Printed in China through Worldprint Ltd.

14 15 16 17 18   10 9 8 7 6 5 4 3 2 1

TITLE PAGE IMAGE

Helping the Wounded by Captain Francis Leopold Mond
(1896–1918) RAF, depicting a blinded soldier in Hospital
Blues being helped by a nurse and was painted to raise money
for the St. Dunstan's Hostel for Blind Soldiers and Sailors.

CONTENTS PAGE IMAGE

The Great Western Railway Medical Fund raised the money
to convert the swimming baths in Milton Road, Swindon into
a temporary Red Cross hospital. It closed in June 1915 when
the military hospital was opened at Chiseldon Camp.

ACKNOWLEDGEMENTS

I would like to thank the following people for their generous
help and for the provision of images. Dr Andrew Bamji,
Hazel Basford and the Powell Cotton Museum, Quex Park,
Birchington UK, Lynette Beardwood and Dawn Waters/
First Aid Nursing Yeomanry, Tony and Linda Chew, Judith
and David Cohen, Alan Cumming, Jennian Geddes, Carol
Gingell/Broadland Memories Archive, Dave Hanmer, Peter
Harrod, Robert Higgins, Sue Light, Rob McIntosh, Sharon
Munday, James Morley, Jon Ratcliffe and Swindon Local
Studies Library, Jon Spence, Abigail Turner/Museum of the
Order of St John, Jane Whisker/State Library of New South
Wales, Paul Williams.

PHOTOGRAPH ACKNOWLEDGEMENTS

Images courtesy of A2Z Military Collectables, pages 6
(left and right), 58 (middle), 59 (far left and middle);
Dr Andrew Bamji, page 1; Broadland Memories Archive,
page 55 (top); Tony and Linda Chew, pages 14 (bottom), 26,
40 (top); Judith and David Cohen, pages 12 (bottom), 25
(top), 34 (bottom), 35, 43 (top); Alan Cumming, page 16
(bottom); FANY (PRVC), pages 7 (top), 10, 40 (bottom);
Garton Archive at Lincoln Christ's Hospital School, page
54 (bottom); Jennian Geddes, page 54 (top); Dave Hanmer,
page 17; Robert Higgins, page 52 (top and bottom), 63;
Imperial War Museum, pages 14 (top), 20 (bottom), 21,
23, 29 (top), 32, 37, 45, 46, 50, 55 (bottom); Library of
Congress, pages 9, 24, 28 (top), 29 (bottom), 30 (top and
bottom), 47, 49; Sue Light, pages 6 (top), 7 (bottom), 15
(top), 16 (top), 34 (top), 36, 58 (bottom), 59; Mitchell
Library, State Library of New South Wales, page 28; James
Morley, page 31; Museum of the Order of St John, page 58;
Otis Historical Archives, National Museum of Health and
Medicine, Maryland, USA, page 19; Powell Cotton Museum,
Quex Park, Birchington UK, pages 8 (top and bottom),
43 (middle and bottom); Preston Digital Archive, page 41;
Army Medical Services Museum, pages 5, 12 (top left), 13
(bottom), 56, 59 (left); Sgt. Sawyer Spence of the Queen's
Westminster Rifles/Jon Spence, page 22 (top); Society of
Friends, pages 15, 38; Swindon Collection, Swindon Central
Library, page 42 (top); Paul Williams, page 3.

Shire Publications is supporting the Woodland Trust, the UK's leading woodland conservation charity, by funding the dedication of trees.

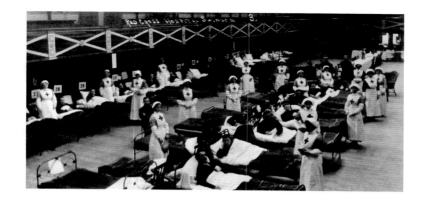

CONTENTS

PREPARING FOR WAR   4

MOBILISATION   10

HEALTH, WELFARE AND WOUNDS   18

THE CHAIN OF EVACUATION   26

HOSPITALS IN FRANCE AND FLANDERS   32

TRANSPORT   38

BRITISH MEDICAL SERVICE ON THE EASTERN FRONT   44

HOSPITALS ON THE HOME FRONT   50

COUNTING THE COST   56

PLACES TO VISIT   60

FURTHER READING   60

GLOSSARY   63

INDEX   64

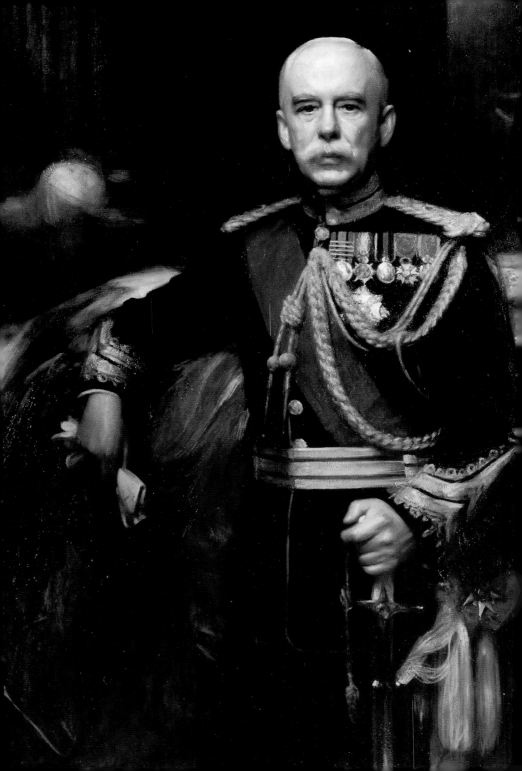

PREPARING FOR WAR

Providing medical services for casualties of the First World War on the Eastern and Western fronts was a complex exercise, without precedent in both scale and nature, and created a huge challenge for all concerned, at home and abroad. Well before Britain's declaration of war on 4 August 1914, official attention was focused on the deficiencies in the way the sick and wounded had been treated in previous wars, especially during the second Boer War (1899–1902), prompting a review of the British Army medical services, directed by Sir Alfred Keogh. As a result, preparations were made to ensure a more efficient organisation in the event of another conflict with sufficient hospital beds for the wounded and enough trained people ready to care for large numbers of patients.

Nursing was the first priority and in March 1902 the army nursing service, which comprised sixty-five serving nurses, was reformed as Queen Alexandra's Imperial Military Nursing Service (QAIMNS), with a reserve corps formed in 1908. In the same year Lord Haldane, the minister of war, inaugurated the Territorial Force Nursing Service (TFNS), which was dedicated to supporting the recently formed territorial force and ultimately replaced its predecessor, Princess Christian's Army Nursing Service Reserve. Those who signed up to the TFNS had to provide evidence of three years' training in an approved hospital. They continued to work in civilian posts and private homes in peacetime, but made an annual commitment to the War Office (WO). The establishment of the Civil Hospital Reserve in 1911 attracted a further 600 trained nurses. The WO then looked to the voluntary sector to boost numbers, and in 1909 Keogh issued the *Scheme for the Organisation of Voluntary Aid,* aimed at providing supplementary support to the TF medical service in case of invasion. A nationwide network of male and female Voluntary Aid Detachments (VADs) organised by county was launched and by April 1911 the British Red Cross (BRC) and the Order of St John (OSJ) had raised 659 detachments between them, with a combined total of 20,000 personnel.

Opposite:
Sir Alfred Keogh
(1857–1936)
was the first
army doctor to
be elevated to
Knight Grand Cross
of the Order of
the Bath. Among
other awards
he received the
Grand Cross of
the Victorian Order
from the King
in the Birthday
Honours for
January 1918.

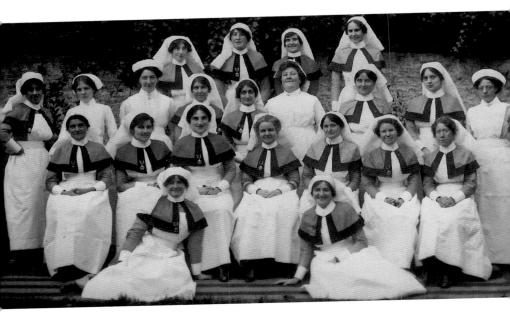

Above: A group of QAIMNS Reserve Force staff, which comprised matrons, sisters and staff nurses under forty-five who could be called upon at short notice. They had to sign a three-year contract and received either an annual £5 retaining fee or, if working, a scaled allowance.

Far right: A QAIMNS Reserve badge.

Right: A TFNS badge, bearing the motto *Fortitudo Mea Deus*, which translates as 'The Lord is my strength.'

In the main the male members worked as hospital orderlies and organised transport whilst their female counterparts undertook food preparation and nursing duties.

Many of those eager to 'do their bit' were middle-class women, and included thirty-four-year-old Mrs Katherine Furse, who joined a London VAD in 1909. She, like other members, was provided with a training course of lectures and introduced to drill and camp life. Among the other units set up in anticipation of war was Mrs Mabel St Clair Stobart's (1862–1954) Women's Sick and Wounded Convoy Corps, founded in 1907, which was officially accepted as a VAD in July 1910. There was also the First Aid Nursing Yeomanry (FANY) founded in 1907 by Captain Edward Baker as a first-aid link between front-line fighting units and the field hospitals, to 'tend British soldiers on the field'. Keogh's re-organisation also included contingency plans for a bed emergency with twenty-five large public buildings — four of them in London and each with capacity for 520 patients

— earmarked for speedy conversion into TF general hospitals. Staffing was organised with ninety-one qualified nurses allocated to every hospital with an additional twenty-one recruited as back-up to ensure a full complement.

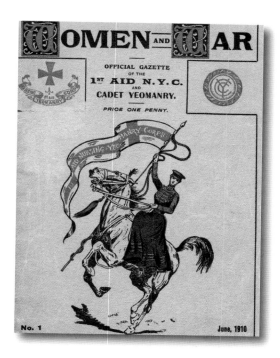

Apart from qualifying in first aid, home nursing, horsemanship, veterinary work, signalling and camp cookery, members of the First Aid Nursing Yeomanry had to buy their own uniform and pay ten shillings enrolment fee.

Below: A group of TFNS nurses, with matron-in-chief Miss Sidney Browne (1850-1941), holding the bouquet. The Florence Nightingale-designed cape was intended to 'conceal the female bosom from the gaze of the licentious soldiery.' The 'T' badge identified the women as members of the TFNS.

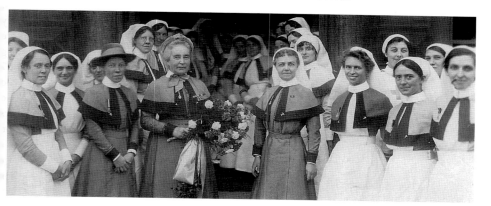

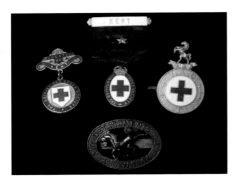

County badges like these, instituted in 1911, were awarded to officers and members of any branches of the British Red Cross or its VADs, including overseas branches, while a connection with the branch was maintained. The badges were worn on the left with either uniform or civilian dress.

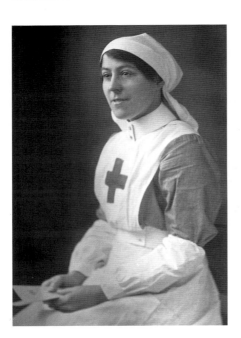

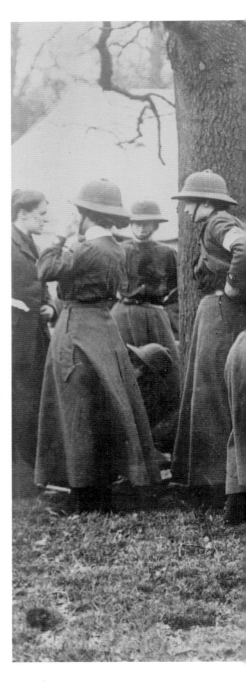

Nurse Hobden, here seen with the red Geneva cross on her apron, worked as a nurse at Kemsing VAD Hospital, Kent, where more than 1,028 wounded soldiers were treated during the war.

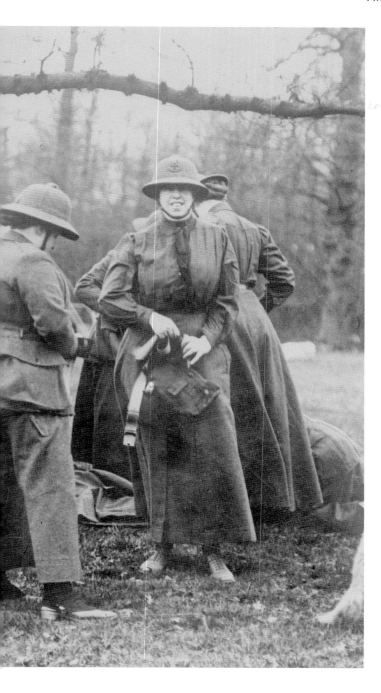

Mrs Mabel St Clair
Stobart's Women's
Sick and Wounded
Convoy Corps was
intended for service
between base and
field hospitals in
the event of a war.
The women trained
once a week in
London and camped
for a fortnight every
year at Studland,
Dorset, where they
learned to pitch
tents, dig trenches
and generally
survive in basic
conditions.

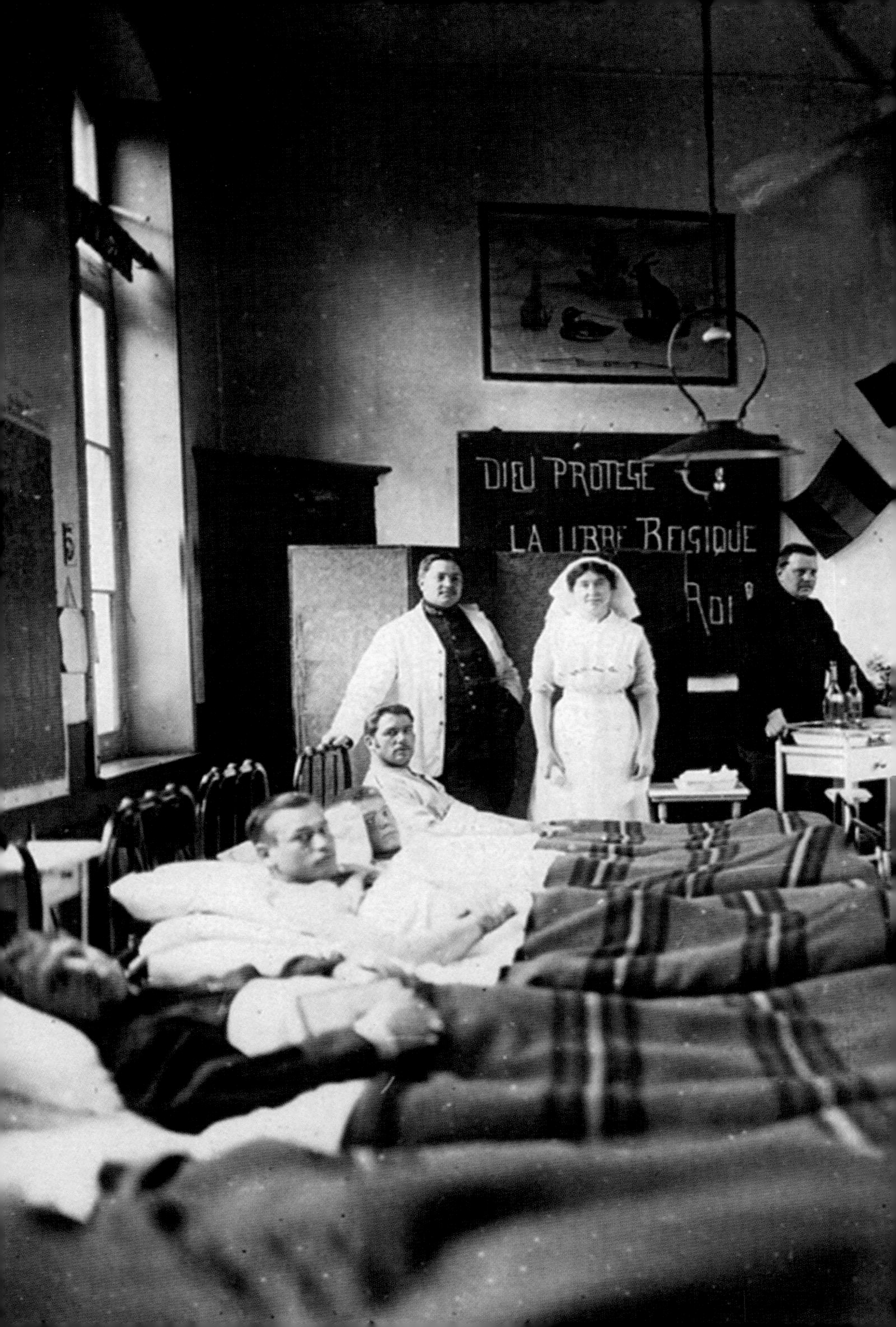
DIEU PROTEGE
LA LIBRE BELGIQUE
ROI

MOBILISATION

WHEN MOBILISATION ORDERS were given following the outbreak of war Keogh was in overall charge of the medical services, Sir Arthur Sloggett was appointed director general of medical services on the Western Front, and Miss Maud McCarthy, QAIMNS, was appointed matron-in-chief for the British Army. The Royal Army Medical Corps (RAMC) immediately deployed around 900 medical officers, 10,000 other ranks and 600 military nurses to France, while Miss McCarthy had 516 regular and reserve nurses under her command. The TFNS had in excess of 2,000 women ready for service and there were 543 male and 1,811 female VADs, with a total of 70,243 personnel, registered with the WO. The BRC and the OSJ combined resources and finances under the umbrella of a new Joint War Committee (JWC) so that voluntary wartime relief work could be administered speedily, efficiently and safely, with the Red Cross name and emblem providing protection. Among the thousands of men and women who responded to the WO call to join the VADs and 'do something for their country' was the feminist and author, Vera Brittain. She joined the VADs as a nurse in 1915 and worked at the 1st London General before being posted to Malta in September 1916. From there, at her request, she was sent to the 24th General at Étaples, France. New members undertook the Red Cross nursing training which included first aid, bed-making and blanket bathing, but in fact VADs – whose nicknames included Very Adorable Darlings and the Starched Brigade – did anything and everything, often in very harsh conditions, frequently receiving a mixed reception, especially from their qualified colleagues. More professional nurses also came forward, and the QAIMNS reserve attracted more than 2,200 women by the end of 1914. By December 1915 it included nurses from Australia and New Zealand as well as 557 highly qualified members of the Queen Victoria Jubilee Institute for Nurses.

Most of the 2,117 TFNS nurses who were mobilised remained in Britain, and like Miss Hastings – who was posted to the 4th Scottish General Hospital,

Opposite:
Interior of Lamarck hospital ward, Calais c. 1914. It soon had 100 beds and between 1914 and 1916 the FANY treated over 4,000 Belgian patients.

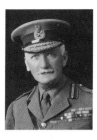

Surgeon-General Sir Arthur Thomas Sloggett KCB CMG (1857–1919), in his British Army uniform.

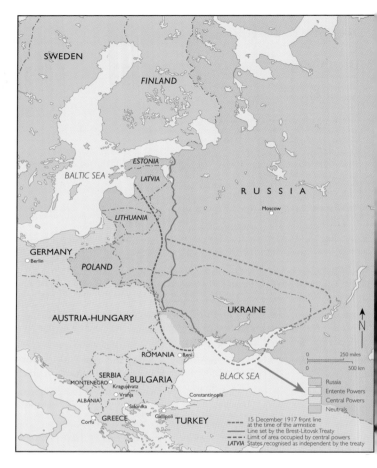

Nurse Edith Cavell (1865–1915) was matron at the Berkendael military hospital in German-occupied Belgium in 1915. She was executed by the Germans on 12 October 1915 for assisting some 200 wounded Allied soldiers to escape to neutral Holland.

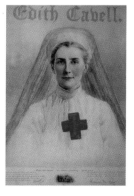

Stobhill – were excited by the prospect and 'dressed, shopped and packed' in eager anticipation of their journey. Some official nurses were already on their way to France and Belgium, welcoming the opportunity to travel abroad, but quite unprepared for what lay ahead. Sister Joan Martin-Nicholson, a Red Cross Sister, found herself ordered to work under the Germans at the Hôpital Militaire in Brussels following their occupation of the city on 20 August 1914, and when Red Cross nurse Kate Finzi arrived at the No. 13 Stationary Hospital, Boulogne in October 1914, she was shocked at being 'part of the tattered remnants of a once-flourishing Red Cross detachment whose energies and equipment alike had been left behind at the enforced evacuation of Ostend'. Other nurses, including Kate Luard,

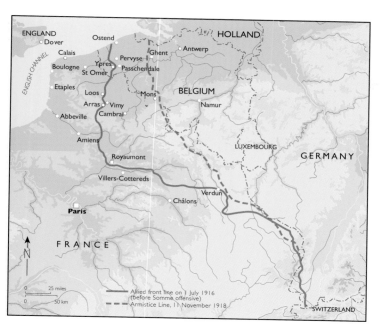

Opposite:
A map of the
Eastern Front.
Left: The
Western Front.

ENGLAND
Dover
Ostend
HOLLAND
Calais
Ghent
Antwerp
Pervyse
Boulogne
Ypres
Passcheridale
St Omer
ENGLISH CHANNEL
Etaples
Loos
BELGIUM
Mons
Arras
Vimy
Namur
Abbeville
Cambrai
Amiens
LUXEMBOURG
Royaumont
GERMANY
Villers-Cottereds
Verdun
Châlons
Paris
FRANCE
N
0   25 miles
0   50 km
Allied front line on 1 July 1916
(before Somme offensive)
Armistice Line, 11 November 1918
SWITZERLAND

Miss Maud
McCarthy
(1858–1949),
QAIMNS. By the
time the Armistice
was signed in
November 1918,
she had about
6,400 nurses under
her command. She
was appointed
Dame Grand
Cross of the Most
Excellent Order
of the British
Empire in 1918.

an experienced Sister in the QAIMNS, initially found themselves with nothing to do. Conversely, the first VAD unit sent out to France in October, under Katherine Furse, was fully occupied from the outset, tending and caring for the wounded in their pioneering rest station in Boulogne. Furse returned to Britain at the end of 1914 to run the VAD department at RC HQ in London, and was appointed commander-in-chief in 1916.

Among the first unofficial organisations to boost numbers abroad was the Millicent Sutherland Ambulance (MSA), established by Millicent, Duchess of Sutherland (1867–1955) for the Belgian RC in early September 1914. She and her team spent six weeks working behind the German lines in Namur, before escaping through Holland. Back in France in October 1914, Sutherland re-established her unit as a temporary 100-bed hospital at Malo-les-Bains, Dunkirk, before moving into tents twelve miles south-west at Bourbourg. With a matron, fourteen nurses, four VADs and two surgeons, the 'Camp in the Oatfield' was operational from May to September 1915, then decamped into huts along the sand dunes at Calais where it became the No.9 RC Hospital (Millicent Sutherland Ambulance) treating British casualties.

The Belgians also happily accepted help from Dr Hector Munro's Flying Ambulance Corps, whose women members included eighteen-

Miss Maynard at the VAD rest station at Abbeville. This was more sophisticated than the one run by Katherine Furse at the Gare Centrale, Boulogne which was housed in 'three trucks and two second-class coaches on a siding', and ministered to thousands of men.

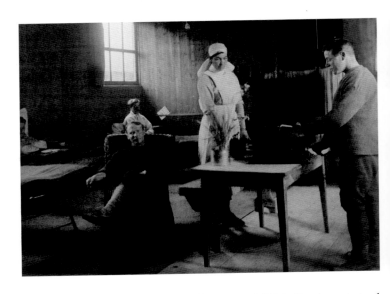

Postcards like these would have encouraged women to join the VADs, and would possibly have been sold to raise funds.

year-old Mairi 'Gipsy' Chisholm and thirty-year-old Elsie Knocker, a trained nurse. Both were ex-motorcycle despatch riders for the Women's Emergency Corps, and their role was to pick up the wounded from close to the firing line, carry them away on stretchers, then tend them in their mobile hospitals. Grace McDougall, née Ashley-Smith (1887–1963), the commandant of the FANY, was firmly turned down by the WO in August 1914, but nevertheless secured an RC pass to go abroad and, despite her lack of any qualifications, spent two months working at a Belgian hospital in Antwerp, attending a constant stream of wounded and dying men, and confronting gangrene for the first time in her life. In late October she got permission to take a FANY corps to France where they had charge of the Belgian Lamarck hospital in Calais. Soon after, a regimental aid post (RAP) was set up not far from the trenches at Ostkirk, and for three months two FANYs, along with battalion doctors of the 3ème Chasseurs-à-Pied, attended the rush of wounded from the front. By October 1914, well-qualified British nurses aged between twenty-eight and forty were being invited by the French government to apply to work for the newly formed French Flag Nursing Corps (FFNC) for a minimum of six months. Amongst the first to work there was Margaret Ripley, a nurse from Guy's Hospital, London, who was at

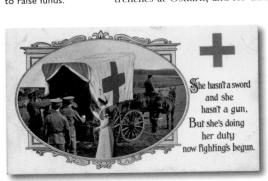

She hasn't a sword
and she
hasn't a gun,
But she's doing
her duty
now fighting's begun.

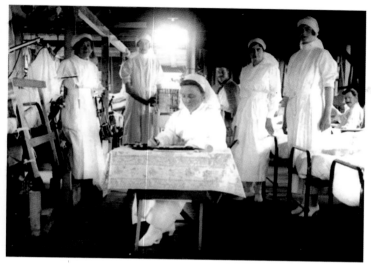

A ward at the Millicent Duchess of Sutherland Hospital. The hospital was administered and largely funded by the duchess, and moved several times before being demobilised in November 1918.

Nurses outside the Queen Alexandra Hospital, Dunkirk, the first of four Friends' hospitals abroad, c. late 1917–18. At least eight hospitals in France and Belgium were staffed by FAU members during the war. Back row, left to right Miss Mary Hardy, Miss Pease, Rachel Wilson, Miss Pease. Front row left to right, Miss Ethel Hay, Miss Molly Evans.

Le Havre and then the Hôpital Militaire de Talence, near Bordeaux. In a postcard sent home in January 1915 she described the place as 'an awful hole' where the patients had no comfort, and was so disheartened by the lack of work and poor conditions that she was eager to leave. Weeks later she was reassuring her mother that she had not been injured in the bombardments in Dunkirk. The Society of Friends established the Friends' Ambulance Unit (FAU) in 1914 and with the support of Sir Arthur Stanley, chair of the JWC, sent forty-three volunteer members abroad on 30 October. En route to Belgium, this pioneering group – which included three doctors, six dressers, eight ambulance cars and several tons of stores – got diverted by the thousands of wounded they encountered in Dunkirk. In the course of three weeks they treated around 3,000 casualties in goods sheds at the station and carried some 6,000 soldiers on board transport ships. The first Friends' hospital, the Queen Alexandra, opened at Dunkirk in March 1915.

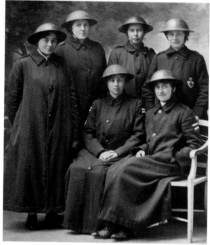

The RAMC, meanwhile, urgently needed more doctors, and those who went to France, like Temporary Lieutenant C. W. Bryan, RAMC, from Queen Mary's, London, were under huge pressure. In November 1914 he was with the No. 14 General Hospital, Wimereux, which had around 600 beds,

Two nurses
with an RAMC
medical officer
and orderlies.

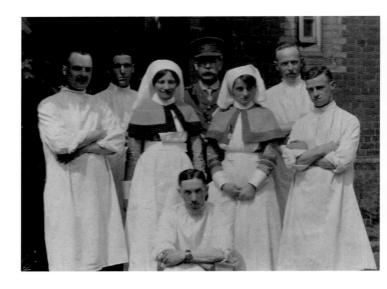

Dr Elsie Inglis, a
qualified surgeon,
became honorary
secretary of the
Scottish Federation
of Women's
Suffrage Societies
in 1909 and was
commandant of
an Edinburgh VAD
when war broke
out. On 3 April 1916
she became the
first woman to be
decorated with the
Order of the White
Eagle, the highest
honour that Serbia
could bestow.

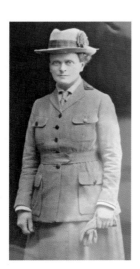

and personally had surgical supervision of 310 cases. He was regularly on
duty for twenty-four hours at a time, with only an hour's break for lunch
and dinner, often sleeping in his clothes, as 'there were so many bad cases
arriving this evening'. To resolve the doctor crisis, the WO progressively
raised the age of eligibility of male practitioners to forty-five for service
abroad, and also sent one hundred 'dressers' – medical students in their
third year – overseas, but they quickly recalled them, realising it was more
important in the long term for them to complete their studies. The
BRC also engaged about 400 doctors for service at home and
abroad, with a further 157 doctors chosen for various positions in
auxiliary hospitals, but had no contract with the JWC. By November
1915 there were 9,626 medical officers abroad, an increase of 2,599
from May, but still insufficient to cope with the huge demands of the
war. Despite this, the RAMC and WO steadfastly rejected the
services of any of the 1,000 or so qualified medical women in
Britain. When former suffragettes Dr Louisa Garrett Anderson
(1836–1917) and Dr Flora Murray (1869–1923) formed the
Women's Hospital Corps (WHC), and offered their complete unit
to the British government, they were resoundingly rejected. But
their direct offer to the French was accepted and between September
1914 and January 1915 they ran a 150-bed voluntary military
hospital from the luxurious Hôtel Claridge in Paris, complete with
operating room, pharmacy and asepticising room. In an about-turn
the RAMC then asked the WHC to set up an eighty-bed hospital at

Wimereux, making it the first hospital to be run entirely by women, and to be officially recognised by the army. The Claridge amalgamated with Wimereux in January 1915 and the combined unit was closed by early March 1915. Keogh was unequivocal in his praise for them and the 'splendid services rendered by medical women in France'.

Edinburgh-educated Dr Elsie Inglis (1864–1917) was also given short shrift by an official who advised her to 'go home and sit still' in response to her plan to set up a female medical corps abroad. Undeterred, and with financial help from the National Union of Women's Suffrage Societies and the American RC, she was welcomed by the French, Russian and Serbian governments. The first unit of her newly formed Scottish Women's Hospitals for Foreign Service (SWH) left for France in November 1914, and included Dr Isabel Emslie (1887–1960) who had also been told by the RAMC that there was 'no use for women doctors in the war'. Another, Dr Dorothea Clara Maude (1879–1959), became one of seven British surgeons at a British field hospital at Ostend and then Antwerp in autumn 1914. When the city was bombarded in October all the patients were transported to Ghent in several London buses, with Dorothea administering morphia to enable the most seriously ill to survive the arduous journey. She returned to the UK by steam packet with some 400 wounded, then returned to France in January 1915. There she responded to an RAMC request for a surgeon at the Sophie Berthelot hospital in Calais. Once they got over the shock of a woman doctor they installed her as an anaesthetist. She then moved again, this time to her uncle's eponymous Maude hospital near Dunkirk.

Dr Hilda Clark (1881–1955), obstetrician, suffragist and Quaker, devoted her medical skills to the victims of war following the devastation of the Battle of Marne. With the support of the Friends' Emergency and War Victims' Relief Committee, she established an emergency maternity hospital at Châlons-sur-Marne in November 1914, followed by a small cottage hospital at Sermaise-les-Bains in March 1915. Eventually the WO was forced to reconsider their attitude towards women doctors and in April 1916 Keogh called for forty women doctors to go out to Malta – in fact eighty-five sailed out in July 1916. At home women doctors were appointed to work in munitions factories attending victims of industrial accident but, despite demands from many quarters, all were denied equal status.

Private Arthur Hamner of the 1st North Staffordshire Regiment, which landed at St Nazaire on 12 September 1914, is believed to have lost a leg and was subsequently discharged from the army.

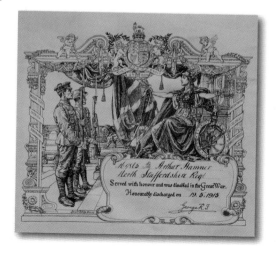

17

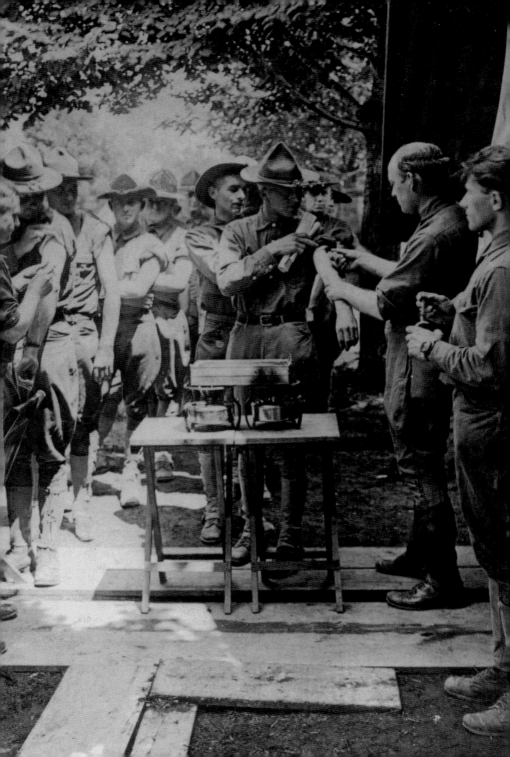

HEALTH, WELFARE AND WOUNDS

First and foremost it was in the military and national interest for soldiers to be fit and well, and disease prevention was one of the most important functions of the medical officers. While vaccination against smallpox was compulsory, inoculation against typhoid (enteric) fever was not. When the British Expeditionary Force (BEF) arrived in France, only 25–30 per cent of troops had any protection against the disease. Doctors like Lieutenant Aubrey Venables, RAMC, battled to provide training in first aid and stretcher-bearing, to take care of sanitation and to vaccinate troops. Despite pressure from groups within the medical fraternity throughout the autumn of 1914, the government sided with the anti-vaccinationist movement and refused to enforce immunisation. But once Lord Kitchener issued an order that only inoculated soldiers could go abroad, take-up improved, and by the end of 1915 an estimated 90 per cent of troops had received the typhoid-specific vaccine, after which the paratyphoid vaccine, TAB, was routinely administered.

The trenches – where the men ate, slept, lived and fought – were hellish places. They were squalid, overcrowded, rat-infested, frequently flooded and perfect breeding grounds for disease. Poor sanitation and lack of personal hygiene were a constant problem, and even though divisional bathing facilities were set up, dirty clothes steam-disinfected and clean clothing issued, around 97 per cent of officers and soldiers still had body lice. 'Greybacks', as they were nicknamed, along with rats, mosquitoes and other creatures, were thought to be responsible for the spread of trench fever, which caused severe headache, shivering, a rash and muscular pain in bones and joints. The symptoms lasted for around five days, sometimes recurring, and left men unfit to resume duties for up to six months. It was not until early 1918 that the link between lice and trench fever was firmly established, and only then were special pits for de-lousing clothes recommended.

Other hazards were trench foot and frostbite, the latter occasionally resulting in gangrene of the toes and amputations. Between November and

Opposite:
Soldiers lining up for typhoid vaccinations c. 1917. A British doctor, Lieutenant Venables, RAMC, wrote that 'If no hitch occurred with the names I did the men at the rate of 200 per hour, i.e. three per minute'.

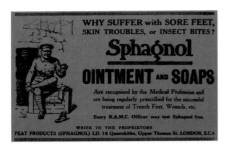

December 1914 alone, 6,378 cases of frostbite were recorded among British troops in France and Belgium, with kilted battalions suffering the added misery of frostbitten knees. Medical officers tried all sorts of futile remedies including wrapping feet in cotton wool or pouring rum into the boots. Once neglect was identified as the root cause, an official programme of care was initiated in January 1915, with men instructed to wipe their boots inside and out with whale oil, to regularly wash their feet in cold water, dry them and then put on fresh socks. Getting such a precious commodity was not easy, and delivering socks to Belgian soldiers in the trenches on the Yser was a task that Pat Waddell, a FANY at Lamarck hospital, carried out under cover of dark and during heavy bombardment. The rest stations run by the Field Ambulances (FA) also helped, rescuing men on the march who were trailing behind their units. Once on the ambulance wagon, boots and socks were removed, and iodine was painted on the sores. After a few days' rest they were fit to return to their regiments.

Soon men were presenting with the devastating injuries of the battlefield, challenging the medical profession to comprehend and treat new physical and mental conditions quickly in order to maintain manpower levels.

Although Mulfords and others were selling vaccines, the majority were supplied by the RAMC's own laboratories, and as a result of their immense campaign, case fatality fell from 12 per cent in 1914 to 6 per cent in 1918, and the incidence of, and deaths from, typhoid (enteric) fever were far lower among British troops than either the French or Germans.

By late 1915, soldiers were limited to spending thirty-six hours in the trenches, and the wearing of gumboots became widespread in wet sectors. Here soldiers of the 12th East Yorkshire are having their feet inspected by the MO in a support trench near Rodincourt, 9 January 1918.

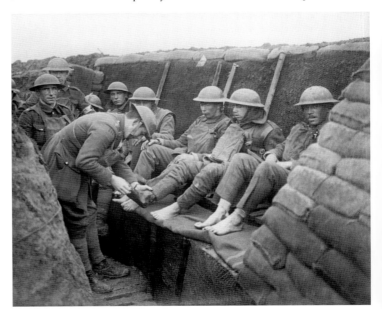

Dr Haden Guest's report in the *British Journal of Nursing* on 31 October 1914, captured the extent of the carnage, reporting that 'every town [in France] was filled with wounded men ... truck loads of wounded... Many of the operations were performed without anaesthetics as no chloroform was available.' According to Dorothea Maude, the chloroform situation was resolved – in Dunkirk at least – in early 1915 when Britain 'rose to the occasion and sent enough chloroform to float a dock and a few voluntary hospitals' such as hers. To enable medical officers to cope with increased numbers of operations, nurses were trained to administer anaesthetics. Less successful was the treatment of soldiers with shell shock brought on by the extreme trauma of war. Symptoms ranged from uncontrollable diarrhoea to unrelenting anxiety, but shell shock was neither understood nor condoned,

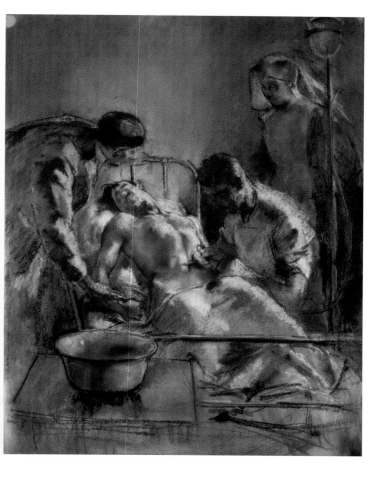

A patient undergoing a saline infusion on a hospital ward in the BRC hospital, Arc-en-Barroise, France, 1915. The treatment was used effectively in Mesopotamia and Sinai, especially in 1916, to treat cholera. The painter Henry Tonks was a surgeon before becoming an artist, and served as an RAMC doctor during the war.

Sergeant Sawyer Spence, Queen's Westminster Rifles, was exposed to mustard gas at close range in France in August 1918, and suffered severe 'burns' to his skin. Back home at Trent Bridge Hospital, Nottingham, he was treated with Burnol Paraffin and made a full recovery.

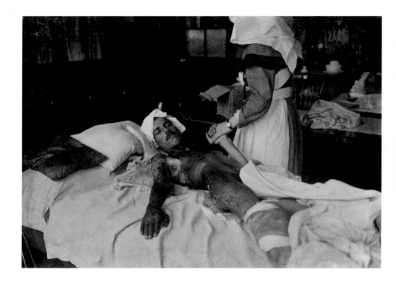

German nurses treating patients, all wearing gas masks. The masks are placed very neatly around the nurses' heads, which may indicate that this was a dress rehearsal.

and elicited little sympathy anywhere, as men were branded cowards and malingerers and sent home.

The 14th Division of the 44th FA were among the first to experience the initial German gas attack at Langemarck on 22 April 1915. The

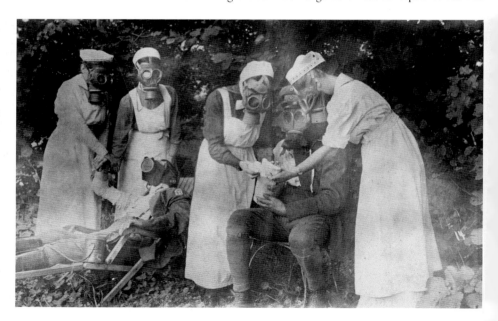

yellow-grey chlorine gas attacked the respiratory system, causing the larynx and bronchial passages to swell up, choking the victim. With no contingency to deal with this new threat, hastily improvised respirators were immediately sent out from Britain, and everyone was drilled 'in the art of tying on, over one's nose and mouth, a black veil containing cotton wool soaked in sodium bicarbonate'. Such emergencies effected advances in treatment: thinning the blood stopped victims panicking, which further depleted the oxygen in the blood. Then came a smoke-hood-type mask, before the introduction of a small box respirator with a flutter valve and a charcoal filter that removed impurities from the air breathed in by the wearer.

More than half the casualties of the early battles on the Western Front were caused by artillery fire, with firearms responsible for a third of wounds, and 5 per cent caused by bayonets, hand grenades and other smaller arms. Soldiers who suffered gunshot wounds to the leg, and the resulting wound-shock, had only a 20 per cent chance of survival in the early days of the war, but by 1917 the new Thomas splint, a metal frame which held and protected a fractured femur, had increased survival rates to around 82 per cent. Once steel helmets became standard issue for forward units, more soldiers survived head injuries. The same could not be said for those with abdominal wounds, especially after a big 'push', when the army surgeon had to consider whether to devote an hour to one man with abdominal wounds and give him half a chance

Doctors placing a patient's broken thigh in traction at a base hospital.

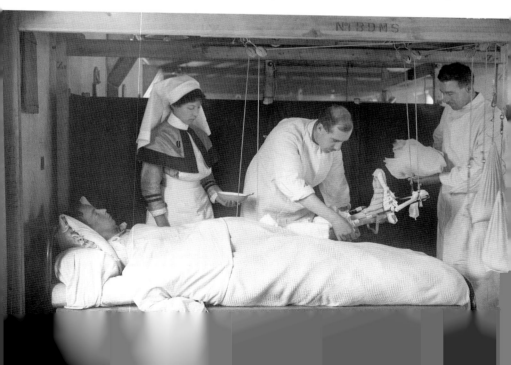

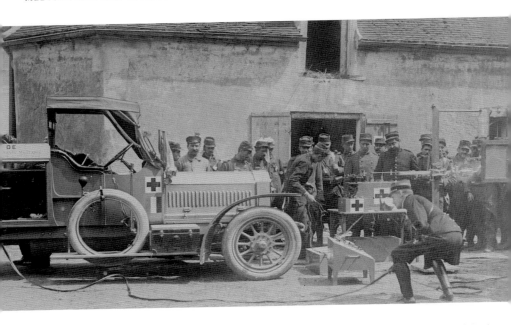

French mobile radiology automobile, c. 1914–15 Mobile x-rays were pioneered by the physicist Marie Curie, who launched a service for the French Army, obtaining suitable vehicles for conversion into 'petite Curies'.

of surviving, or give an hour to others with severe wounds to the head, limbs etc, and save at least three lives. Given this choice, many medical officers put abdominal cases to one side to die. Nursing personnel had to watch carefully for any signs of the sweet, mouse-like smell that characterised gas gangrene, caused – as Sister Kate Luard described – by 'the presence in the wound, in the deep tissue, of a very virulent microbe'. Amputations were all too common and frequently failed to arrest progress of the disease, but by 1916 the practice of 'delayed primary suture' had been adopted, which improved survival rates.

The initial lack of x-ray equipment hampered the medical staff, and worried nurses like Sybil Cooke whose diary entry in October 1914 reflected her concern: 'The government are terribly slow, and in the delay lives and limbs are being sacrificed.' In January 1915 there were still only two mobile x-ray cars in the British Army, and the SWH sent their first travelling x-ray motor ambulance to the front in August 1915, working under the RC. In contrast, the British-funded Urgency Cases Hospital, established in March 1915 in a disused military barracks near the French lines at Bar-de-Luc, had an excellent x-ray unit. In one instance Mr Forsyth, the médecin-en-chef, was able to remove a large fragment of shrapnel casing from a soldier's shoulder within half an hour of seeing the x-ray. X-rays also made it possible for a skilled surgeon to use the bullet extractor, which the *British Journal of Nursing* described as an 'ingenious instrument'.

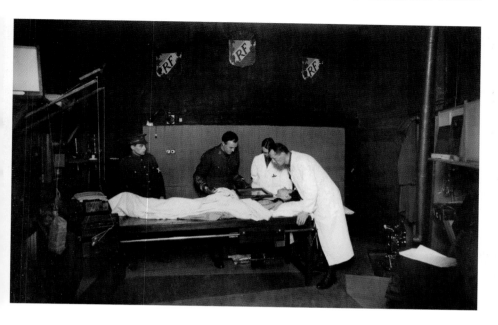

By 1917 blood transfusion was firmly established in the casualty clearing stations as a routine measure and by the end of the war, shock and its management were far better understood. The Millicent Sutherland Hospital was recognised for its efficient use of the revolutionary Carrel-Dakin wound-irrigation treatment, using an antiseptic solution containing sodium hypochlorite. Even old infected wounds responded and healed more quickly, and the general condition of the patient improved almost immediately. Drs Murray and Garrett Anderson made their own contribution by adopting the use of BIPP, a paste made of bismuth, iodoform and paraffin, for treating wounds, while Liverpool surgeon, Miss Frances Ivens (1870-1944), analysed a series of cases of anaerobic infection, and collaborated with the *Institut Pasteur* in pilot trials of gas gangrene antiserum.

Military x-ray machine at the No.1 BRC, Duchess of Westminster Hospital, Le Touquet.

CONDY'S FLUID

The Pioneer Oxidant,

" AT THE FRONT "

CONDY'S FLUID disinfects and cleanses Wounds, Sloughing Wounds, Burns, Ulcers, Gangrene, Bedsores, &c.; prevents Tetanus and Wound Infections. It establishes and maintains odourless aseptic conditions without causing irritation, all its effects being benign, soothing, and wholesome.

Hydrogen Peroxide, the other available oxidant, is very painful as a dressing owing to the acid added to it as a preservative.

CONDY'S FLUID is free from potassic permanganate, the incautious use of which has caused deaths (16 Coroner's Inquests) and many minor injuries.

Proper directions for 150 uses with every bottle.

CONDY'S FLUID WORKS,
65, GOSWELL ROAD, LONDON.

From May 1917 the Carrel-Dakin procedure became standard practice in hospitals, but medical journals at home were still advertising disinfectants like Condy's fluid.

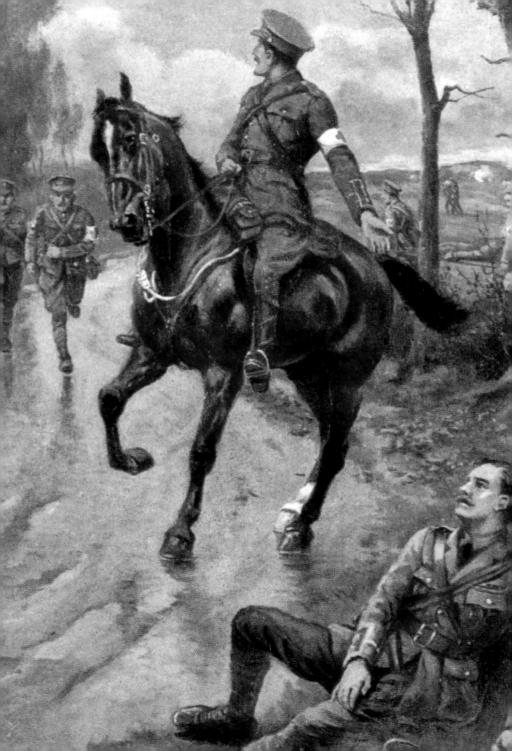

THE CHAIN OF EVACUATION

S URVIVAL DEPENDED on prompt medical intervention, and it became evident early on that pre-war planning for getting men to the field hospitals was woefully inadequate. The RAMC chain of evacuation began within two to three hundred yards of the front line at the RAPs, which were set up in small spaces such as communication trenches and derelict buildings. Often places of death and confusion, the lack of light added to the mounting apprehension. The walking wounded struggled to make their way to the RAP, while more serious cases were carried by comrades or even a stretcher-bearer. The single regimental medical officer (RMO) was a qualified doctor, and typically only had experience of domestic general practice, and knew little or nothing about war wounds. If he was lucky he had two trestles on which to treat the wounded, but treatment was limited to administering pain relief, an anti-tetanus injection and applying a basic dressing at best. The RMO could only cope with about twelve casualties at a time, and in the heat of battle sometimes enlisted the help of the regimental stretcher-bearers, who were trained in first aid. It was not until July 1915 that some uniformity in the method of treatment was established with the publication of *Memorandum on the Treatment of Injuries in War: Based on Experience of the Present Campaign*.

Once stabilised, casualties were transported as quickly as possible to the advanced dressing stations (ADSs), which were provided and run by the FAs, non-vehicular mobile front-line medical units. Located further away from the front line, they utilised ruined buildings, underground dug-outs and bunkers: anywhere that afforded some protection from shell fire and air attack. Each FA had ten officers and 224 men, and was divided into three sections, which in turn had thirty-six stretcher-bearers, an operating tent and six bell tents, complete surgical outfit, dressing, drugs, and cook's apparatus. In the autumn of 1915 some FAs had trained nurses posted to them. Travis Hampson – a medical officer with No. 20 FA in France in 1914

Opposite:
An official RAMC postcard c. 1914–15, with officers wearing caps rather than helmets, and depicting a sanitised view of the battlefield. Such cards may have been produced for propaganda purposes or to raise funds.

Stretcher-bearers
carrying wounded
soldiers into a
first-aid station.

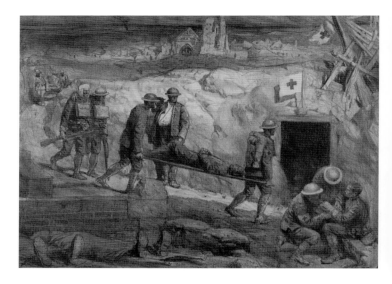

– recalled how every doctor had a surgical haversack and a mysteriously
named 'monkey box' which the medical orderly carried on a shoulder strap
and which contained 'a fair variety of dressings and instruments.' But he
also mentioned the all-important 'medical comforts ... not a vast amount,
as these things are liable to disappear mysteriously!' which included a bottle
of brandy, a dozen half-bottles of champagne, condensed milk and meat

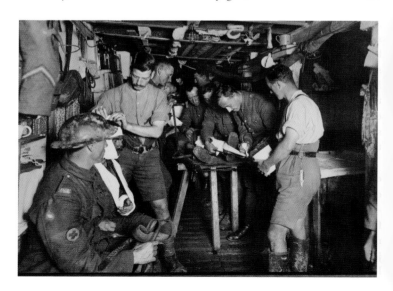

Medical staff
attending the
wounded in the
ADS on Hill 60,
c. 1917–18.

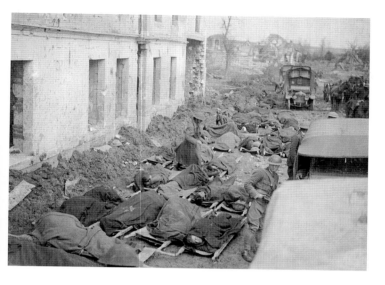

Stretcher cases waiting to be moved by motor and horse-drawn ambulance from the advanced dressing station at Blangy near Arras, April 1917, following the first battle of the Scarpe.

extracts. With so many casualties, and to avoid congestion, three different 'posts' were set up, one for walking wounded, one for the collecting and another for relaying men. Teams of stretcher-bearers were posted over miles of ground, or trenches, and the wounded were passed along these lines, often in very dangerous conditions, with many daytime transfers of urgent cases halted because of direct enemy fire. For Walter Bentham, with No. 8 CC RAMC, 23 August 1914 at Mons was 'his baptism by fire … simply awful to see and hear the shells bursting around us'. A system of carrying stretchers shoulder-high, four bearers to a stretcher, was, as far as stretcher-bearer Edward Munro was concerned, less tiring than two carrying with slings, but either way, the bearers were exhausted at the end of the day. Munro wrote of the hazards of getting a footing on greasy and slippery tracks cut up by shells, and of how even the most severely injured soldiers did not complain about the discomfort they endured.

Red Cross transport carrying the wounded in the Forêt de L'Aigle, September 1914.

The next stage was the casualty clearing station (CCS) – known as clearing hospitals until mid-1915 – but getting the wounded there from the ADS, usually several miles away, was often a dreadful journey undertaken by ambulance, lorry or even railway. The lack of

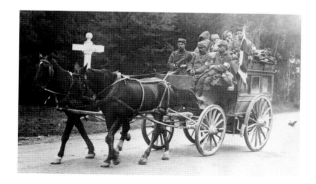

A wounded soldier taking bandages from a Red Cross dog's 'kit'. Dogs were trained to carry medical supplies and to seek out casualties in no man's land.

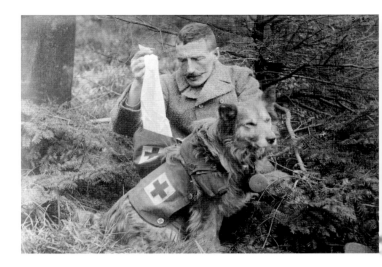

motorised ambulances in the early stages of the war meant the FAs relied heavily on horses for transport, requiring a large establishment of animals to work the rubber-tyred ambulance wagons and support vehicles. The CCSs were the first static units that a casualty encountered, and were set up in convents, schools, factories or even sheds at large railway junctions. Nurse Kate Finzi worked at one in France in late October 1914, where 'ten beds and a number of sacks of straw form the main equipment. Planks, supported by two packing cases are the dressing table.' The operating theatres typically had one table and one steriliser for instruments, perhaps three jugs of sterilised lotions and a travelling table. Dressings went unsterilised,

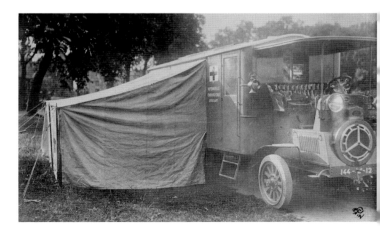

A French mobile operating ambulance, c. 1914–15.

wards lacked trolleys and dressing tables, and empty petrol cans served as receptacles for soiled dressings. Even the introduction in early 1915 of basic trestles on which to place stretchers proved to be an absolute boon to patients and nurses. So too did the comforts provided by the BRC which included-bed linen, socks and nightwear.

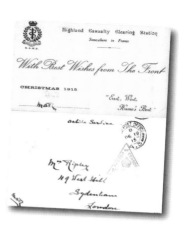

By the spring of 1916 some of the CCSs were as well equipped as the best of the general hospitals, and the majority were a mix of huts and tents with only a minority of beds in buildings. As more surgery was undertaken, x-ray equipment became an integral part of the set-up, with an x-ray lorry attached to a group of CCSs. By spring 1915 triaging had been introduced, whereby casualties were divided into three treatment priority categories. It soon became clear that nurses could play a valuable role in the CCSs, and once authority was received on 29 October 1914, five senior QAIMNS sisters were posted to No.3 Poperinghe and five to No.6 Merville. The first battle of Ypres highlighted the impossibility of five nurses coping with an influx of between 1,200 and 1,500 casualties in twenty-four hours, and by March 1915 the first of several emergency staff reserve systems was in place. In January 1915 tours of duty were restricted to three months, a reflection of the stress of work and the dangerous conditions experienced by nurses like Edith Appleton, working at No.3 CCS Hazebrouck. On 18 April 1915 they had over 600 through their hospital, and two days later she wrote the following:

Nurse Ripley's postcard home, Christmas 1915, gave her mother no clue as to where she was posted in France. Like many nurses, she was sent to a temporary hospital near the firing line, details of which had to be kept secret. The Highland CCS (No.51) was actually based at Lillers until January 1916.

...Frantic day from 7 a.m. to 10 p.m. one long rush of badly wounded being admitted, three train loads have been evacuated. It is a wicked war. Officers and men – many so blown to bits that they just come in to die, many straight to the theatre for amputation of limb or limbs – or to have their insides – which have been blown out – replaced – and made a little more comfortable for the few hours left to them.

As the number of casualties grew, especially from the battle of the Somme in July 1916, when there were between 16,000 and 20,000 casualties on the first day of the offensive, so the need for experienced staff increased, and by August 1916 selected CCSs had as many as twenty-five nurses on the staff. CCSs moved many times, frequently at very short notice and often staying only two or three days at their next stop. Casualties were then moved even further back from the front line to the base hospitals, from where they stood a reasonable chance of survival.

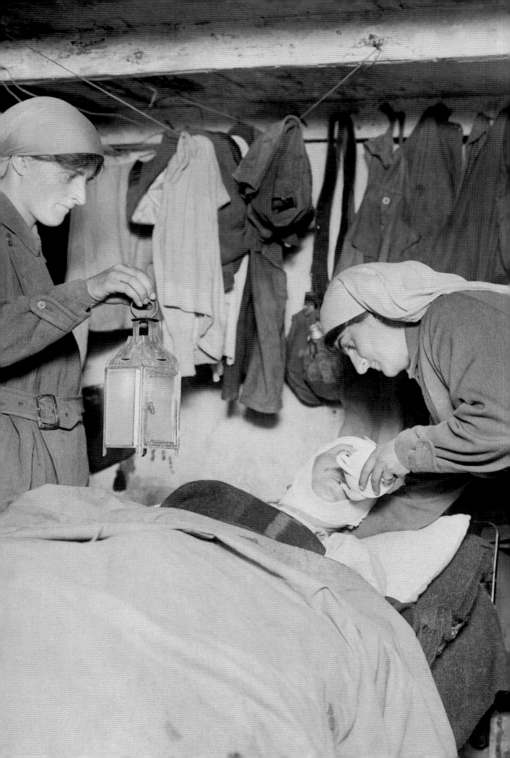

HOSPITALS IN FRANCE AND FLANDERS

THE RAMC ran two types of base hospitals on the Western Front: stationary — which rarely moved — and general, which were mostly situated in or near large towns and coastal ports, with huge numbers concentrated at Boulogne and Étaples. Eventually totalling around sixty-one, most were supported by voluntary organisations, notably the RC, who had jurisdiction for six hospitals in Paris, while the St John Ambulance brigade ran their own 520-bed hospital at Étaples. Air attacks during May 1918 almost completely destroyed the hospital, killing eleven patients and nine members of staff. As the army expanded in 1915, so too did the accommodation, almost doubling in capacity from around 500 beds. At the end of 1915 a typical general hospital, which was divided into medical and surgical sections, was staffed by about thirty-four medical officers, seventy-two nurses and 200 auxiliary RAMC staff, with around 1,000 tons of medical and ordnance stores. Unlike in Britain, where Keogh had buildings on standby for conversion, the French authorities were slower to respond, and other than at the ports, many of the early complexes were huge tented units. These were eventually replaced by wooden huts, with tents added as and when required, expanding capacity from 700 to 1,200 beds. The lack of basic facilities took some getting used to, as Olive Dent — a VAD at one of two general hospitals on the racecourse at Rouen — recorded in her diary: '... no hot water, no taps, no sinks, no fire, no gas-stoves ... only six wash-bowls for the washing of 140 patients...' An ability to improvise, was, as she remarked, essential.

The BRC and the WO received many offers of help in the form of voluntary hospitals, and while these came to play an important role in supplementing the RAMC units, none were allowed to provide medical aid to the troops without official authority. The French and Belgians took an entirely different view and accepted assistance from innumerable British men and women who were determined to 'do their bit'. In 1914, Mrs Stobart established the Women's National (Imperial) Service League, to facilitate

Opposite:
Mairi Chisholm, holding the light, while the Baroness de T'Serclaes (née Elsie Knocker) attends a wounded Belgian soldier at Pervyse, their third advanced first-aid post, 6 August 1917. Both women were awarded the Military Medal in 1917, when Mairi was also given the Belgian Queen Elizabeth Medal with Red Cross.

Tented accommodation overseas. The nurses' quarters are in the round tents.

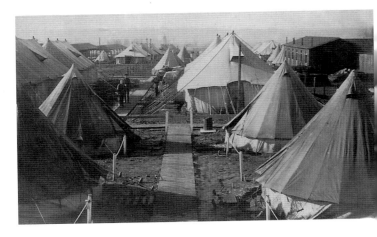

A ward in the Duchess of Westminster Hospital, No.1 BRC, which was based in Le Touquet from October 1914 to July 1918. The author J. R. R. Tolkien was treated here for trench fever.

women's war service both at home and abroad. At the invitation of the Belgian RC she established her first hospital with six medical women and ten nurses in a concert hall in Burchem, Antwerp, with Dr Florence Stoney

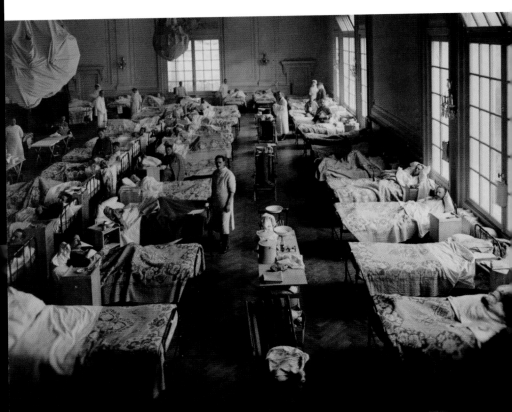

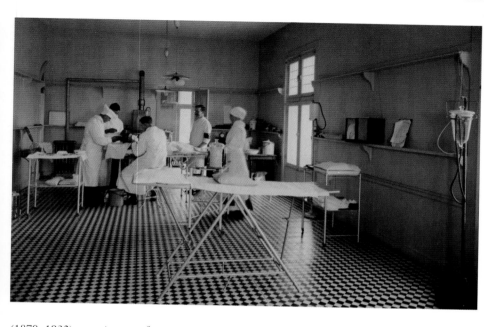

(1870–1932) – a pioneer of x-ray treatment at the Royal Free Hospital, London – appointed médecin-en-chef and radiographer. Within five days the 135 beds were full, and remained so until 8 October when the hospital came under bombardment for eighteen hours. Stoney and her staff managed to get the wounded moved to safety in less than thirty-five minutes, later escaping before being evacuated to Britain. Within a month they were operational again, this time at the Anglo-French Hospital No.2, created in the sixteenth-century Château Tourlaville in Cherbourg. Lacking the basic requirements for a hospital, they generated their own power from a stream in the grounds to supply the x-ray plant and provide light. In March 1915 Stoney was one of the first women doctors to be accepted for full-time work under the WO and Keogh appointed her as head of the radiological department to the Fulham Military Hospital.

Determined to save more lives, Mairi Chisholm and Elsie Knocker parted company with Dr Munro's corps, and by mid-November 1914 had set up a first-aid post in the cellar of a ruined house in Pervyse, Belgium, within fifty yards of the trenches. Undeterred by the perpetual cold, dirt, discomfort and danger, they worked tirelessly treating wounded soldiers as well as those suffering from frostbite, pneumonia and bronchitis before being shelled out in March 1915. They were soon officially attached to the third division of the Belgian army, and with British-donated funds opened up a new aid post near Avecappelle on 11 April 1915 and continued their

The operating theatre at the Duchess of Westminster Hospital, No.1 BRC, Le Touquet, France.

exhausting work. In March 1918, after three and a half years of 'packed incidents', they were gassed by mustard and arsenic shells, and retired from the front.

Lady Dudley's voluntary hospital for the Australian RC in Wimereux was one of many located in small hotels and, despite there being a shortage of beds, Maud McCarthy, who visited on 3 November 1914, was particularly impressed by the way it was being run. Pacifist Harold Reckitt was another individual who worked independently for the Allies. His joint venture with Lady Johnstone, wife of the British minister at The Hague, became the 100-bed Hôpital Militaire V.R.76 at Ris-Orangis near Paris, and operated between September 1915 and October 1918, with the wounded arriving by hospital train direct from the front line.

From January 1915 until March 1919, the SWH ran a 100-bed unit hospital in the Abbaye de Royaumont, near Asnières, about twenty-five miles behind the front line. The damp and insanitary building was transformed under the command of the chief medical officer, Miss Frances Ivens, and given the French RC seal of approval. Between Royaumont and an ancillary CCS opened at Villers-Cotterets, the two units treated a total of 10,861 patients, while a number of canteens were set up in 1917 catering for French soldiers in transit.

Hove, Sussex, War Hospital Supply Depot. Around 553,000 cases and bales of stores, amounting to more than 84,000 shipping tons, were despatched overseas during the war, a process that was made especially difficult when submarines became involved in 1917.

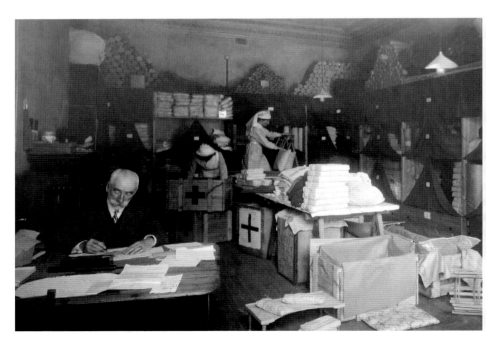

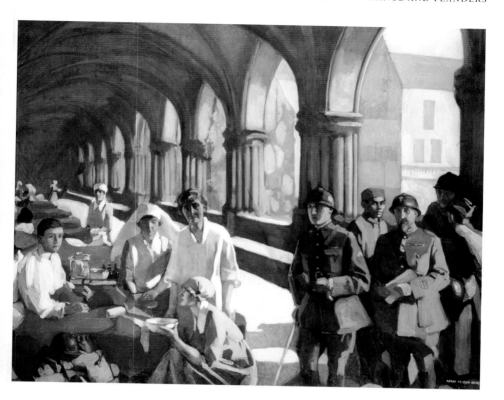

Nurses selected from the register of the National Union of Trained Nurses staffed the Urgency Cases Hospital at Bar le Duc, and in the course of only six months, from March 1915, admitted 838 patients, and performed 364 operations. The unit moved in September 1915 to the Château of Faux Miroir, Revigny, where the ambulance train from the Argonne stopped every day to deliver wounded men. In February 1916 wounded troops began to arrive from Verdun, with 236 admitted between 11 February and 10 March alone. The workload was arduous and the toll on the nursing sisters was huge but, despite requests for leave in June 1916, only those who were sick were given any time off.

Within months of the Americans entering the war in 1917, the medical assistance that they had promised the BEF began to arrive in France. The first base units took over six British general hospitals, where half of the 1,100 or so nurses were stationed. The QAIMNS staff were withdrawn, but as the hospitals found themselves short of staff, temporary help was provided by VADs until reinforcements arrived from America.

Miss Frances Ivens, in the white coat, inspecting a French patient in the Scottish Women's Hospital set up in the cloister of the Abbaye de Royaumont. The artist, Norah Neilson-Gray (1882–1931), worked there as a VAD nurse from 1914–18. The hospital expanded to accommodate 600 men and became the largest continually operating voluntary hospital in France.

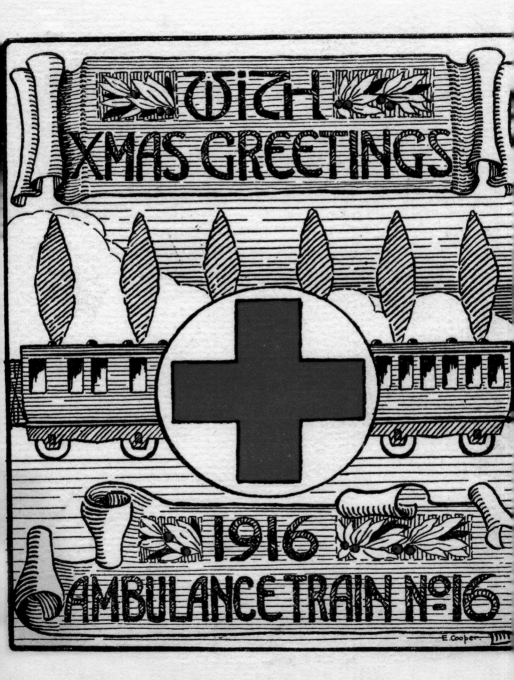

TRANSPORT

TRANSPORTING PATIENTS from the CCSs to the base hospitals, evacuation ports and home was a precarious job which involved horse-drawn and motor ambulances, ships, boats and barges, as well as specially adapted ambulance trains. The pre-war decision made by Brigadier-General Sir Henry Wilson, director of military operations, not to send motorised ambulances with the BEF to France in August 1914, went against the consensus view in medical circles and quickly proved to be a disaster. Horse-drawn ambulance wagons were unable to cope with the volume of wounded from the battle of Mons, from 23 August 1914, and reports soon reached home of soldiers being left to die, or being taken prisoner by the Germans, for lack of transport. To rectify the situation Lord Kitchener called for public donations towards the purchase of vehicles, and with the BRC motor ambulance department established, *The Times* appeal raised enough money by mid-October for the RC to purchase 512 ambulances. Other appeals and funds paid for the maintenance of the vehicles. But the insufficiency of ambulances still worried Sloggett and Keogh, who described them as 'the sheet-anchor of medical services in forward areas and ought to be used much closer to the front'. The WO subsequently ordered that every army corps should have one motor ambulance convoy which included fifty ambulance cars capable of carrying four to six patients, and by 6 November 1914 there were around 250 vehicles available in France, with more arriving daily. In just six months in 1915, the driver for No.1 BRC VAD unit at Abbeville took 1,677 cases to hospital and hospital ships. Many of the 2,500 drivers who served with the JWC, and those of the voluntary organisations, were women, even though it was a hazardous occupation and haunting experience. Under Lilian Franklin, the FANY ran the Calais Convoy for the British between January 1916 and the Armistice, with the unit described as 'a bracing caravanserie' comprising twenty-two drivers plus mechanics, twelve ambulances, three lorries and a motorcycle.

Opposite:
A Christmas greeting card from The Friends' Ambulance Unit, which began running ambulance trains in 1915.

39

An official RAMC postcard showing a motor and horse ambulance on the Western Front.

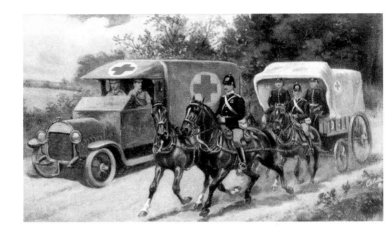

Mairi Chisholm and Elsie Knocker of Dr Hector Munro's Flying Ambulance Corps arrived in Ghent on 26 September 1914, and spent the first two months ferrying seriously wounded men in the two ambulances at their disposal. When hundreds of casualties arrived by train from Antwerp on 3 and 4 October, the two women worked tirelessly day and night to get them to hospital. The FAU also staffed and ran three French ambulance convoys, each of twenty-two vehicles, for the *Sections Sanitaires Anglaises*. One driver, Olaf Stapledon, recalled how 'Occasional shelling afforded the required sense of danger ... then there was the night-driving without lights, on roads pitted with shell-holes ... Every bump called forth cries from the suffering men within the car.' The No.14 convoy alone carried

Two FANY drivers posed with a BRCS ambulance, northern France or southern Belgium, 1914–18. The First World War uniform included a cloth cap instead of a pith helmet, which was dropped because it did not fit into the cabs of the ambulances.

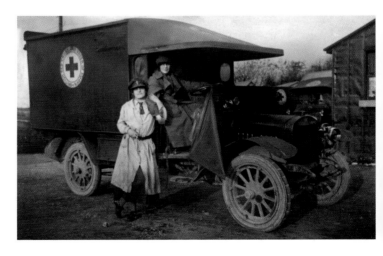
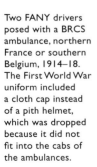

50,960 wounded during the course of the war, traveling 402,734 miles. Horse-drawn vehicles continued to play an important role throughout the war, but carrying the seriously injured across otherwise inaccessible muddy and heavily cratered ground required a team of six horses rather than two.

The lack of ambulance trains was yet another contentious issue early on in the war, precipitating heated questions in the House of Commons. Equipment for six had been sent to France with the BEF, but lacked engines or rolling stock. While the early ambulance trains were created in assorted French railways goods wagons and carriages, with capacity for 800 casualties, Travis Hampson, an RAMC medical officer, recorded having to utilise empty supply wagons to move patients in mid-August 1914. The alternative was to put them in 'ordinary trucks improvised to take stretchers and some of the usual vans with straw on the floor'. The wounded could be neither fed nor treated on board, and had to wait until they reached a hospital for attention. Train arrivals were often unexpected, and when 1,000 were suddenly due at the BRC dressing station at Abbeville station on 15 May 1915, VAD Eleonora Pemberton nearly panicked and had to borrow extra orderlies from another unit to help cope. In readiness, her routine included making gallons of cocoa, uncovering everything in the surgery, preparing lotions, getting the primus stove going, and later assisting the medical officer with dressings.

The No.12 was the first properly designed British ambulance train to arrive in France in November 1914, and was fitted out with beds down either side of the carriage to maximise capacity and enable the medical staff to attend to patients. Some trains had operating theatres, although the movement and the cramped conditions made surgery a difficult task.

Concerns about overcrowding of the French and Belgian rail network, and the delays this caused, inspired the BRC to follow the French example and utilise barges on the waterways, enabling men to be transferred direct to hospital ships. Although the journey was slow, it was more comfortable than either train or motor ambulance, and enabled nurses to attend and dress wounds regularly. Staff Nurse Mildred Rees, QAIMNS Reserve, who spent five months on the No.4 ambulance flotilla on the Somme in 1916, also emphasised how much the wounded 'loved the barge and it does them the world of good', reinforcing the importance of non-medical care. Nurses from the FFNC also staffed two hospital barges, which

Poster for a fund-raising theatrical evening in Preston, Lancashire. All manner of events including concerts, flag days, and exhibitions were held up and down the country to raise money for ambulances and to support hospitals at home and abroad.

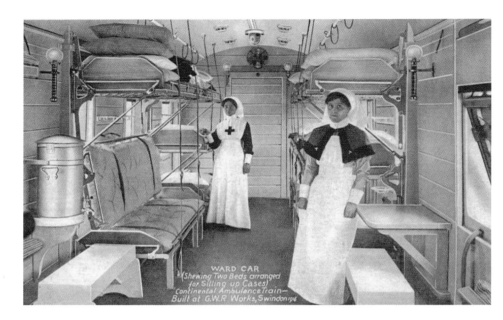

WARD CAR
(Shewing Two Beds arranged
for Sitting up Cases)
Continental Ambulance Train—
Built at G.W.R Works, Swindon 1914

The inside of an ambulance train carriage, built at the Great Western Railway works, Swindon.

The interior of a hospital barge showing the cargo hold converted into a functioning ward. Makeshift hand-operated lifts enabled stretchers to be lowered below, and rudimentary ventilation was provided in the roofs. Each barge had at least one QAIMNS sister, an RAMC orderly and auxiliary help, and shared an RAMC medical officer with other barges.

transported the seriously wounded along the canal from Adinkerke, Belgium, to Bourbourg, France.

Most hospital ships were requisitioned and converted passenger liners, like the White Star Line RMS *Aquitania*, which did two years' service from 4 September 1914. This was the largest of the ships and on one

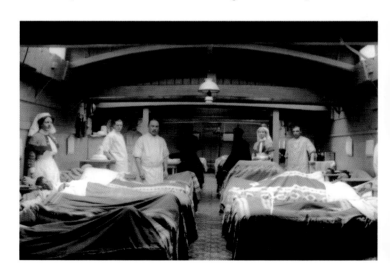

journey from the Dardanelles she had nearly 5,000 patients on board, requiring twenty ambulance trains at Southampton to distribute them to various hospitals in Britain. The risk of mines and torpedoes was very real and it was pure fortune that fewer than thirty-five people lost their lives when the *Asturias* was hit in March 1917. Mary Stevenson, a Queen's nurse, survived and later wrote 'I thank God with all my heart that our patients (between 900 and 1,000) had been taken off a few hours before.'

The small regular force of Queen Alexandra's Royal Naval Nursing Service was boosted by 200 reservists during the war, providing care at fifteen naval hospitals and on nine hospital ships, and by 1916 the FAU had two ambulance ships, the *Western Australia* and the *Glenart Castle,* for which they provided the staff of orderlies and non-commissioned officers under the RAMC doctors and nursing sisters.

On arrival at a British port, the wounded were transferred to a home service ambulance train and transported to one of the 196 receiving stations, as near to home as possible.

A commemorative glass plate showing the hospital ship *Braemar Castle*. On 23 November 1916, when carrying 400 sick and wounded, it hit a German mine and became the second hospital ship to go down in the Aegean Sea within a week.

A Kent VAD transport badge.

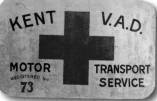

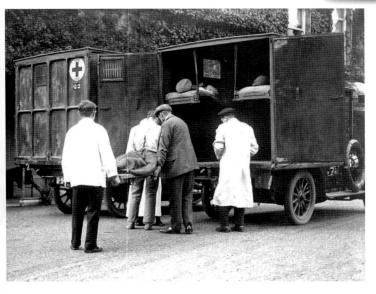

Between November 1914 and December 1915 the men of the VAD Kent 43, Folkestone, assisted with the detraining at Shorncliffe station and transport to local hospitals of fifty-eight convoys of wounded British soldiers, totalling about 4,700 men.

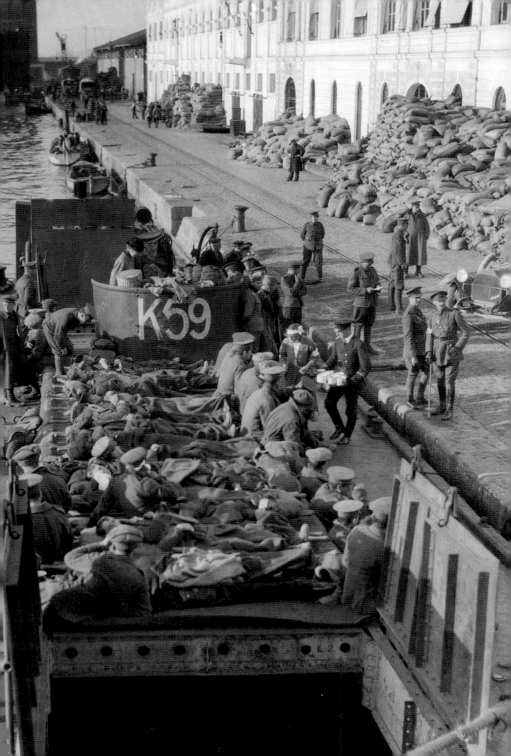

BRITISH MEDICAL SERVICE
ON THE EASTERN FRONT

T HE PROVISION and effectiveness of medical services for the BEF
and Allied troops in the other theatres of war, including Gallipoli,
Salonika, East Africa and Mesopotamia, was very varied, and was never
as well organised as it became on the Western Front. Official reports
describe catastrophes reminiscent of the Boer War, due largely to
managerial problems and the exclusion of medical officers at the planning
stage. Only later on – when the Western Front chain of evacuation model
was adopted – did matters improve. Evacuating the wounded was the
priority, but the army was inexperienced in moving casualties by sea
and the numbers predicted – between 10,000 and 11,000 for the April
1915 landing – were grossly underestimated. Within three weeks
nearly 20,000 were brought back to the base in Alexandria, and some
250,000 casualties were evacuated from Gallipoli by January 1916, but
initially there were no established hospitals, and the single Australian
dressing station was totally overwhelmed. To overcome the bed crisis,
civilian hospitals were commandeered for British and Anzac troops, but
conditions were sometimes terrible, as Sister Eveline Vickers Foote,
based at the 17th General Hospital Alexandria, recorded, with patients
crowded into marquee tents, and instruments boiled in a small saucepan
because there was no steriliser. Despite this situation, Keogh refused
to give Lady Howard de Walden (1890–1971) permission to establish a
hospital in Egypt in 1915, maintaining that everything was well in hand.
Ignoring this, she went with a matron, eleven fully qualified nurses,
stores and equipment to Alexandria where she set up the convalescent
hospital No.6 in a mansion near Ramleigh. There they tended thousands
of post-operative men sent from the authorised hospitals, freeing up
beds for the next batch of wounded. Even when the bed crisis was
resolved, there was still an acute shortage of medical and nursing staff,
despite the numbers of VADs and nurses who arrived from Britain
and the Dominions.

Opposite:
British sick and
wounded aboard
a motor lighter in
Salonika harbour,
awaiting transfer
to a hospital ship.

45

An ambulance wagon in the mud in Gully Ravine, Gallipoli, following the storm of November 1915. Only mules and horses could traverse the peninsula's rough terrain. Artillery wagons were also used, often driven by the nursing Sisters.

Other medical services lacked equipment, and whilst the East Lancashire Fusiliers had three FAs, only one was complete while the other two were still lacking in essentials three weeks later. The stretcher-bearers had an equally bad time, for with no wheeled transport available they had to carry the wounded across miles of very rough terrain. Many men suffered from trench foot and frostbitten feet from standing for days in icy water in the Gallipoli trenches in the winter of 1915, while others had contagious enteric diseases. And as Private Clarence Whitaker, RAMC, said of five months on Suvla Bay, 'it was hell on earth ... we were always under shell fire'. Transporting the wounded away from the field of battle was a nightmare as Captain L. B. Cane, RAMC, reported on 14 August 1915: 'from the beginning the hospital ships were quite insufficient to deal with such thousands...' They were also inadequate, with one Australian vessel, the *Seang Choon*, described by Colonel Begg, the deputy director of medical

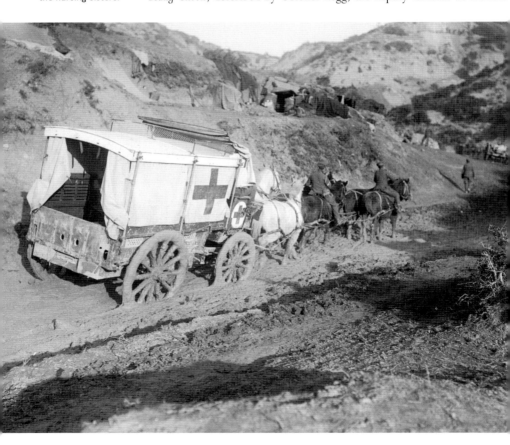

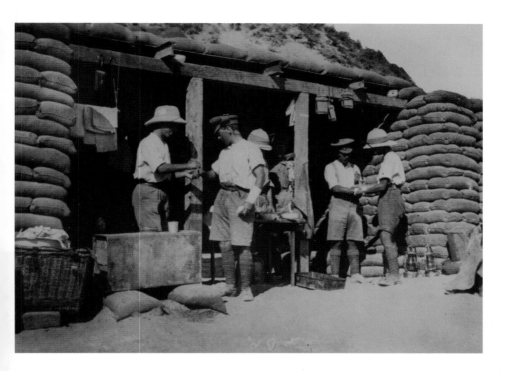

The British Expeditionary Force in the Egyptian area Advanced Field Ambulance dressing station on the Gaza front, 1917.

services of 2nd Anzac division, as 'totally unsuitable for carrying seriously wounded cases … grossly overcrowded … no operating room available'. Working in such conditions exerted a huge strain on the nursing staff, who found it difficult to promote wound healing in the intense heat on board ship, and sometimes resorted to dressing wounds under chloroform to reduce the trauma.

An urgent need for medical support for troops and civilians in Serbia resulted in the establishment of the Serbian Relief Fund (SRF) in London in 1914. From November 1914, with some sponsorship from the SWH, the SRF helped maintain five units. The first, a 600-bed typhus hospital outside Skoplje, was administered by Leila, Lady Paget (1881–1958), the second was the eponymous Cornelia Lady Wimborn unit, while the third was set up by Mrs Stobart, who arrived in Kragujevatz, Salonika in April 1915. This was housed entirely in tents which she described as 'mostly double-lined … specially made to order, by Messrs. Edgington of Kingsway, for wards, staff, X-ray, kitchens, dispensary, lavatories, baths, sleeping, etc., etc., with camp beds and outfit'. Typhus, typhoid, scarlet fever and diphtheria were rife, and the workload was so great that more equipment and manpower were sent from home. A series of roadside dispensaries to provide free medical aid for the peasants followed in June 1915, and within four weeks treated more than 2,500 patients, many of whom travelled miles by ox-cart. Each unit had a female doctor, two nurses, a cook, a 'handy' chauffeur and an interpreter and cost £1,000 to run for three months, so that expansion was dependent on funds raised at home.

The remaining SRF hospitals, Mr Wynch's 1st and 2nd British Farmers' Ambulance Units, were specially organised and equipped to deal with either wounded soldiers or infectious diseases like typhus. Dr Dorothea Maude joined the second unit near Pozarevac in July 1915 as one of four staff physicians treating sick Serbian civilians in outpatient clinics and administering anaesthetics in a nearby camp hospital. After a spell back in Britain she rejoined her uncle on Corfu in March 1916 at the second of his hospitals, and moved with it to Salonika six months later and finally to Vodena before returning home in 1917. In addition, the SRF sent nurses to Mrs Hardy's hospital at Kragujevatz, and a contingent of nurses to the typhus colony formed by Lady Paget at Skoplje. The Royal Free Hospital, London, excluded from the London territorial hospital scheme, was sanctioned by the BRC to send out a unit to Serbia, and the Anglo-Serbian Hospital, or eponymous Berry Mission, was set up at Vrnjatchka Banja. The first unit, comprising six doctors and twelve orderlies, was sent out on 29 October 1914 and, despite being set up in a factory building lacking proper sanitation, managed to care for 800 severely wounded men. The second unit served from January 1915 to February 1916 and treated military and civilian patients.

Dr Inglis, whose first SWH unit was well settled in France, was also welcomed by the Serbs, and her second unit set out for Kragujevatz – where typhus was raging – in late 1914. Here they encountered Mabel Grouitch's St John Ambulance unit and Flora Sandes, who was working with them as a nurse, and who subsequently became the only British woman to serve as a front-line soldier with the Serbian army. By the end of March 1915 the SWH were in charge of three hospitals, nursing 550 beds. When Bulgaria attacked Serbia in October 1915, Dr Inglis, who had joined them in May, and most of her staff stayed on, as did Lady Paget and her team. Inglis's hospital was taken over by the Germans, and she was put in charge of the only prisoner-of-war hospital in the town. She was interned until February 1916 when she was sent home, only to go abroad again months later. In August 1916 the Russian government asked the British for four medical units, two of which were supplied by the JWC, the other two by the SWH. Dr Inglis took seventy-five female staff and two orderlies, and set up hospital at Medjidia, Romania, before being asked to establish a field hospital under canvas at Bulbulmick with just twelve staff. Very quiet periods were interspersed

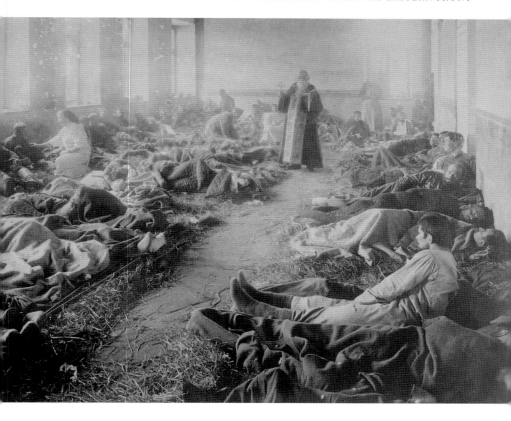

with 200–300 wounded arriving within a few hours, and the staff kept themselves ready to retreat at a moment's notice as the danger increased. November 1916 found them in Ismaila, Russia, where they came under the control of the Russian RC, joining a third retreat in January 1917. They stayed in Reni, Romania, until September, when the unit rejoined the Serbian division in the village of Hadji Abdul, Bessarabia.

Meanwhile, having served in France, Dr Isabel Emslie became a member of the Corps Expeditionnaire d'Orient, which the French sent out to Salonika in October 1915 to help the suffering Serbian army and civilians. She travelled with the SWH Girton and Newnham unit, and served in a SWH hospital at Salonika before being ordered, in summer 1918, to command the SWH hospital in a disused regimental barracks in Vranja. What she found was an indescribable stench: 'people lying on the floor, on straw and on beds without mattresses.' The operating theatre was 'ghastly, and nothing that I had imagined approached it in frightfulness'.

Nurses and doctors tending patients while a priest holds a Russian Orthodox service in a makeshift hospital near the Augustow forest, Suwalki (now Poland), in c. 1914–1915.

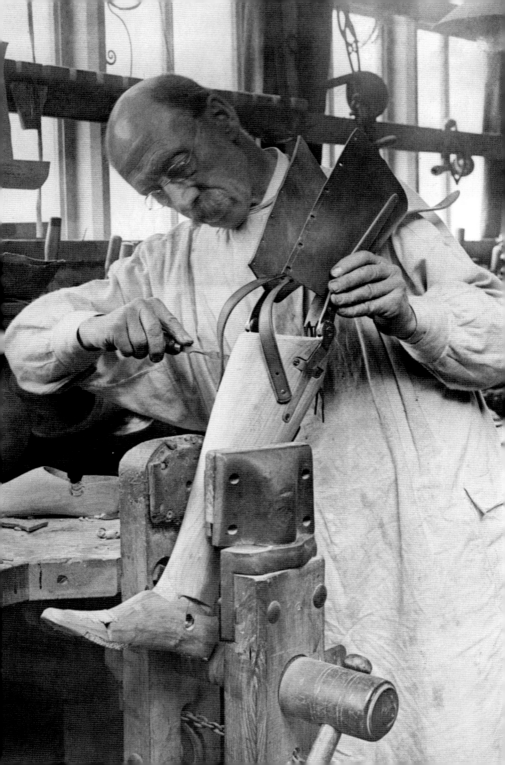

HOSPITALS ON THE HOME FRONT

TREATING WOUNDED and sick men at home quickly became the aim, but following the arrival of the first flood of casualties in Britain on 8 September 1914, it became evident that the existing military hospitals could not meet the demand for beds. Immediate expansion was essential and one solution was to build hutted wards in the hospital grounds, which happened at the 955-bed Royal Victoria, Netley, one of the largest and most important hospitals. By mid-November 1914, the huts – which were 'light, airy and well ventilated ... warmed by slow-combustion stoves ... amply supplied with water ... with admirable sanitary arrangements' – were ready to accept 300 of the planned 500 British and Indian soldier patients. L. Ethel Nazer nursed many Sikhs and Gurkhas and described the arrival of one batch:

> Five out of the last twenty were hand and arm wounds and these walked in; the other fifteen were all heavy stretcher cases; some had six or eight wounds from shrapnel and three were badly frost-bitten; one has since died, another developed tetanus and several amputations have had to be done; all the wounds are horribly septic on arrival but it is surprising how quickly they clean up with regular dressing and attention.

Tents in the grounds of Trinity College, Cambridge, functioned as the 1st Eastern TF hospital while public buildings ranging from schools and churches to stately homes were converted into military hospitals. The home service of the FAU were also involved in the establishment and running of four hospitals in Britain, two of them in Quaker premises. But the most remarkable wartime hospital was Endell Street Military Hospital, created in the former St Giles Union workhouse, London, which Dr Louisa Garrett Anderson and Dr Flora Murray of the WHC were asked to operate by Keogh. Run by women for men, it opened in May 1915 with Murray as doctor in charge, Anderson as chief surgeon, and a staff comprising around fifteen doctors including visiting specialists, thirty-six nurses, eighty

Opposite:
Making an artificial leg for a wounded serviceman at Roehampton Hospital, Surrey, 1917. From an initial twenty-five patients the hospital expanded, and by June 1918 there were 900 beds and a waiting list of 4,321. Some 240,000 men had limbs amputated during the war.

The No.1 operating theatre at Beaufort Military Hospital, which was Bristol Lunatic Asylum (Glenside) before conversion by the War Office. The war artist Stanley Spencer was stationed as a medical orderly there.

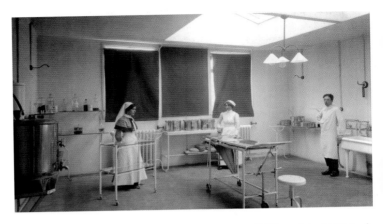

The newly built HM Stationery Office and Stores in Stamford Street, London, was converted and opened as King George Military Hospital in October 1915. By 1917 it had around 1,900 beds, reputedly the largest military hospital in the UK.

women orderlies and a small army of support staff. The original 520 beds soon increased to 573, and by 1919 had a further three auxiliary hospitals attached to it, raising the bed capacity to 800. As Murray recalled in 1920 'it gave women an exceptional opportunity in the field of surgery'.

Many of the diseases suffered by soldiers required specialised care, and hospitals and units were established across the country to treat specific conditions, including venereal diseases, typhoid fever, consumption, dysentery and septicaemia. Among the hospitals set up to treat men suffering from psychological trauma or shell shock was Craiglockhart hydropathic hospital, Edinburgh. It opened in 1916 and was renowned for having the war poets

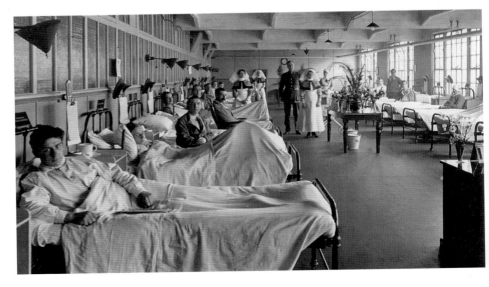

Wilfrid Owen, Robert Graves and Siegfried Sassoon among its patients. By the end of the war the army had dealt with 80,000 cases of shell shock, four-fifths of whom were never able to return to military duty. Soldiers whose faces were seriously disfigured by bullet wounds and flying shrapnel benefited from the groundbreaking reconstructive plastic surgery pioneered by Dr Harold Gillies (1882–1960), who became interested in this branch of medicine while volunteering with the BRC in France. Gillies returned home in 1915 and began work reconstructing the faces of disfigured troops at the first plastic surgery unit set up in the Cambridge Military Hospital, Aldershot, and then at The Queen's Hospital for Facial Injuries, Frognal, Sidcup. He developed procedures involving extensive bone, muscle and skin grafts to restore their appearance, allowing men to go on to live a full life as civilians. For VAD nurse Judy Stokes, treating the men 'as one would any other' helped their mental recuperation, and she was overwhelmed by the spirit they displayed.

The establishment, in June 1915, of Queen Mary's Hospital, Roehampton by Mary Eleanor Gwynne Holford, was yet another pioneering achievement. Her ambition 'to start a hospital whereby all those who had the misfortune to lose a limb in this terrible war, could be fitted with the most perfect artificial limbs human science could devise'. Besides limb-fitting services, patients had access to training opportunities and help with finding employment.

Auxiliary hospitals provided additional beds, with some 250 run by the JWC, and from March 1915 so-called 'convalescent' homes – which effectively kept recovering soldiers under military control – provided

The Royal Brighton Pavilion complex, with its 'oriental domes and charming gardens', was one of three locations in Brighton chosen to house Indian patients. It had a caste committee appointed so that dietary arrangements and religious festivals could be observed. Photograph taken c. 1915.

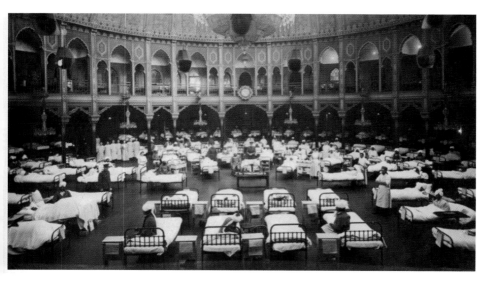

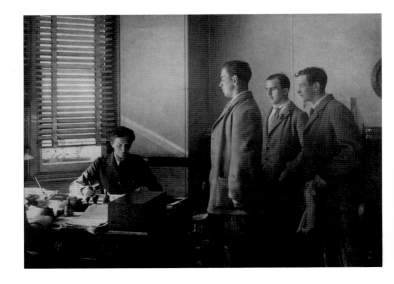

Dr Flora Murray discharging patients from Endell Street Hospital, c. 1915–19. When it closed at the end of 1919, more than 24,000 British, Canadian and Colonial troops had been treated there.

accommodation for 13,384 patients. Many were in stately homes and 655 servicemen enjoyed the hospitality of the Gascoignes at Lotherton, Barwick-in-Elmet, Yorkshire, between November 1914 and March 1919, with all the costs, including conversion, maintenance and staffing, met by the owners. Added to these were hospitals in Hampshire and Berkshire run

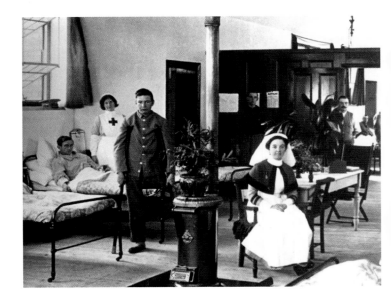

Over 45,000 men were treated at the 4th Northern General Hospital in Lincoln, which was created in the buildings and grounds of what is now Lincoln Christ's Hospital School. It had beds for forty-one officers and 1,126 other ranks.

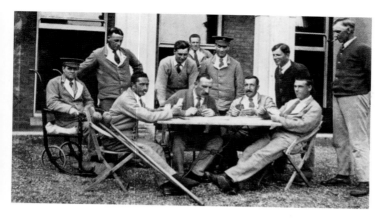

Patients at Brundall House VAD Hospital, Norfolk, were also entertained with concerts, stage plays and boat trips on the River Yare. Their standard issue blue flannel suits and red ties prevented them breaching rules which banned visits to the local pub, c. 1915–18.

by the Canadians, including one at Cliveden, the home of the Astors. By early September 1914, wounded soldiers at the principal UK military hospitals, including Aldershot and Netley, had access to the eponymous Almeric Paget Massage Corps, which began with fifty staff. After being given WO recognition in early 1915 it became the professional model for all massage and electrical departments in convalescent depots throughout the UK and treated an average of 200 patients a day. In January 1917 military masseuses were asked to work overseas, with fifty-six serving in France and Italy up to and beyond the Armistice.

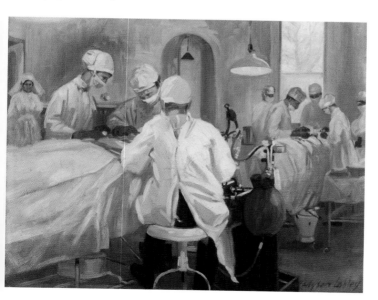

Two operations in progress in 1918 at the purpose-built Queen's Hospital for Facial Injuries, Frognal, Sidcup, Kent. The unit moved here from Cambridge in June 1917 and under Gillies's direction became the central military hospital for facial and jaw injuries. Painting by J. Hodgson Lobley, an official war artist for the RAMC.

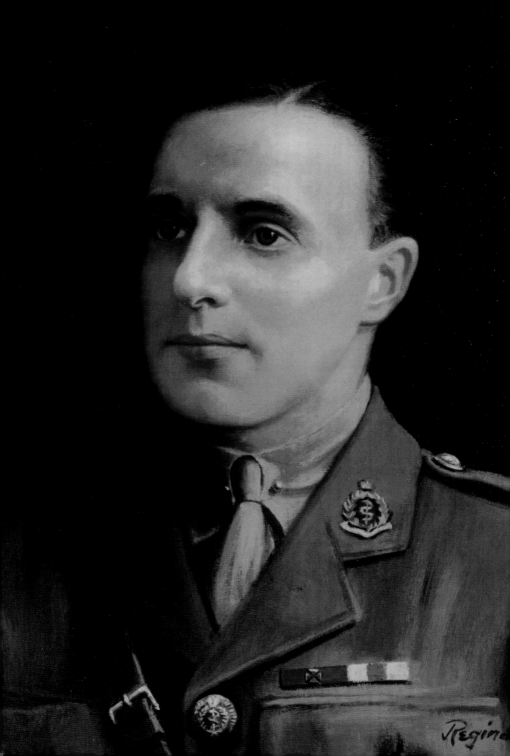

COUNTING THE COST

OFFICIAL FIGURES produced in the 1920s gave the toll of British soldiers wounded during the conflict as 2,272,998, of whom 64 per cent returned to duty, 8 per cent were invalided out, and 7 per cent died of their wounds. This puts into context not only the human cost but also the remarkable and unprecedented contribution, achievements and sacrifices of the men and women who provided medical services in the First World War, at home and abroad. In 1918, the RAMC was greater in size than the whole of the BEF of 1914, with 13,000 officers and 154,000 other ranks, but the corps suffered the loss of 743 officers and 6,130 soldiers. Members were regularly mentioned in dispatches, and a large number of awards were made, at home and abroad, for gallantry to men of all grades. These included 499 Distinguished Service Orders with twenty-five bars, 1,484 Military Crosses with 184 bars, three Albert Medals, 395 Distinguished Conduct Medals with nineteen bars and 1,111 Meritorious Service Medals with one bar. Of seven Victoria Crosses awarded to medical personnel, the highest accolade was paid to Captain Noel Chavasse, the only man to be awarded the Victoria Cross twice in the First World War. For his actions during the war, Surgeon Lieutenant Arthur Martin-Leake became the first man to receive the bar to the Victoria Cross, having received the latter in 1902. By the end of the war the RAMC had sixty-one hospitals on the Western Front and many more at home, whilst the BRC had established 1,786 auxiliary hospitals and staffed ambulances, hospital trains and motor launches to evacuate the wounded to hospitals. They had also provided 90,000 VADs, including 23,000 volunteer nurses, who had helped wounded and sick soldiers at home and abroad. The war had shown the potential of the Red Cross volunteer base, but also highlighted the need for strengthened cooperation between societies. As a result the International Federation of Red Cross and Red Crescent Societies was formed in 1919 to coordinate future peacetime activities.

Reflecting on the work of the women under her command, Maud McCarthy wrote of 'the wonderful thoughtfulness of the nurses in the midst

Opposite:
Noel Godfrey
Chavasse MA, MB,
B.Ch. (1884–1917)
was attached to
the 10th Battalion,
Liverpool Scottish,
and died of
wounds received
while treating
the wounded
during battle. He
was awarded the
Victoria Cross in
1916 for saving
twenty badly
wounded men
under heavy
fire and was
posthumously
awarded a bar
to his VC, for
his courage and
self-sacrifice
during action at
Wieltje, Belgium.

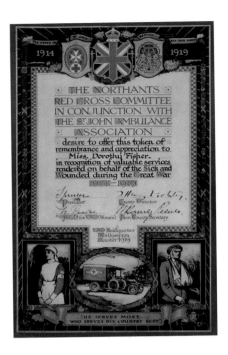

VAD certificate awarded to Miss Dorothy Fisher.

Some members of Durham St John Ambulance brigade were among the staff killed in the air attacks on the SJA hospital in Étaples in 1918. Twenty-seven VAD hospitals were set up in County Durham, and seventeen in Northumberland.

Made of silver, the second class Associate Royal Red Cross was added in 1915 and was conferred upon women members of the nursing service, irrespective of rank. The date 1883 on the obverse refers to the year the first class RRC was instituted.

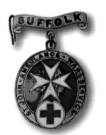

of their arduous duties' and of their concern for the relatives of wounded and dying soldiers. She called attention to 'the great courage and absolute disregard of self shown by nurses carrying on their duties calmly and collectedly with complete self-forgetfulness during a heavy enemy bombardment' and praised the untrained members for their work. In all at least 400 women doctors worked in Malta, Egypt, Salonika and India during the war, while in France they served with Queen Mary's Army Auxiliary Corps, created in 1917, but none of them were permitted to serve on the front line. Even though there was nothing that a woman doctor could not do during the First World War, it did little to improve their career prospects in peacetime. They had to wait until the Second World War to be commissioned into the British Army.

The Society of Friends, which included non-Quakers, made a significant contribution at home and abroad, and in France and Belgium alone the number of personnel had grown from forty-three in 1914 to 640 in November 1918. By then the SWH had fourteen units established in six different countries, with over 1,000 women serving, and included Scottish contingents as well as women from various parts of Britain, Ireland, Canada, Australia and New Zealand. In all about 450 members of the FANY worked as nurses and ambulance drivers on the Western Front with the Belgian, French and British armies.

Many individual medical women received recognition from the Allied countries whom they served, notably Mrs Stobart, Elsie Knocker, Mairi Chisholm and Miss Ivens while FANYs were awarded seventeen Military Medals, one *Legion d'Honneur* and twenty-seven *Croix de Guerre*. Among the nine decorations that Grace Ashley-Smith received was a

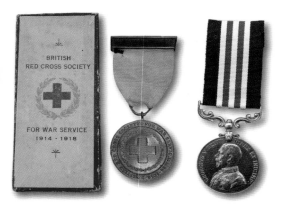

Far left and middle: The BRC medal was awarded to between 41,000 and 42,000 members and VADs who had served at home between 4 August 1914 and 31 December 1919. Eligibility requirements were at least 1,000 hours of unpaid service, or 500 hours in the case of ambulance drivers and bearers. The motto on the reverse reads *Inter Arma Caritas*.

Left: The Military Medal was established by George V in March 1916 and was awarded for acts of gallantry to fifty-five nurses of QAIMNS and the TFNS, and to 3,002 members of the RAMC, along with 199 bars.

rosette to the Mons Star, making her one of the few women to be so honoured. The French government awarded the *Médaille de la Reconnaissance Française* to all the British nursing sisters who served with the FFNC.

Below: Victory parade, 19 July 1919. Miss McCarthy, centre, to the right of the officer; Ethel Becher, matron-in-chief, War Office, on his left; Miss Sidney Browne, matron-in-chief, TFNS, immediately behind the right shoulder of Miss Becher. Some 200 QAIMNS members lost their lives while on active service.

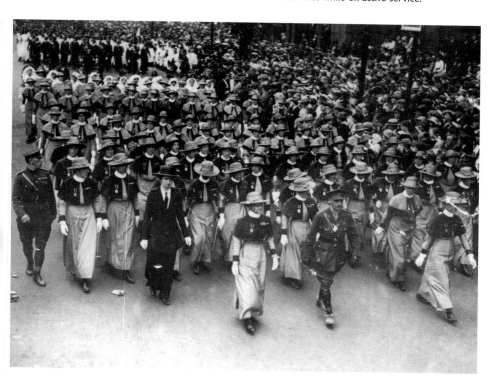

PLACES TO VISIT

Army Medical Services Museum. Keogh Barracks. Ash Vale, Aldershot, GU12 5RQ. Telephone: 01252 868612. Website: www.ams-museum.org.uk
The Imperial War Museum London, Lambeth Road, London, SE1 6HZ. Telephone: 020 7416 5320. Website: www.iwm.org.uk
The British Red Cross Museum and Archives. Website: www.redcross.org.uk
The website also includes very useful links to other nursing organisation collections and other relevant institutions which could be of interest.
National Army Museum, Royal Hospital Road, Chelsea, London, SW3 4HT. Telephone: 020 7881 6606. Website: www.nam.ac.uk.
The Museum of the Order of St John, St John's Gate, St John's Lane, Clerkenwell, London, EC1M 4DA. Telephone: 020 7324 4005. Website: www.museumstjohn.org.uk.
Covers the history of St John's Ambulance in the First World War.

FURTHER READING

Ashworth, Tony. *Trench Warfare, 1914–1918: The Live and let Live System*. Pan, 2000.
Atkinson, Diane. *Elsie and Mairi go to War. Two Extraordinary Women on the Western Front*. Arrow, 2010.
Bergen, Leo van. *Before My Helpless Sight: Suffering, Dying and Military Medicine on the Western Front, 1914–1918*. Ashgate, Farnham, 2009.
Blair, John. *Centenary History of the Royal Army Medical Corps 1898–1998*. 2nd ed., iynx, 2001.
Bowser, Thekla. *The Story of British VAD Work in the Great War*. 1925; Imperial War Museum reprint, 2009.
Brittain, Vera. *Testament of Youth. An autobiographical study of the years 1900 –1925*. Virago, 2004.
Chisholm, Mairi, and T'Serclaes, Elsie. *The Cellar-House of Pervyse*. A&C Black, 1917.
Cowen, Ruth. *A Nurse at the Front: The First World War Diaries of Sister Edith Appleton*. Simon & Schuster, 2013.
Crewdson, Dorothea (ed. Richard Crewdson). *Dorothea's War. The Diaries of a First World War Nurse*. Weidenfeld & Nicolson, 2013.
Crofton, Eileen. *The Women of Royaumont – A Scottish Women's Hospital on the Western Front*. Tuckwell Press, 1997.
Gruber von Arni, Eric, and Searle, Gary. *Sub Cruce Candida: A Celebration of One Hundred Years of Army Nursing 1920–2002*. QARANC Association, 2002.

Hallett, Christine. *Containing Trauma: Nursing Work in the First World War.* Manchester University Press, 2009.

Harris, Kirsty. *More than Bombs and Bandages: Australian Army Nurses at Work in World War I.* Big Sky Publishing, NSW, Australia, 2012.

Harrison, Mark. *The Medical War: British Military Medicine in the First World War.* Oxford University Press, 2010.

Horton, Charles (ed. Dale Le Vack). *Stretcher Bearer! Fighting for Life in the Trenches.* Lion Hudson, 2013.

Krippner, Monica. *The Quality of Mercy — Women at War. Serbia 1915–18.* David & Charles, 1980.

Lee, Janet. *War Girls: The First Aid Nursing Yeomanry in the First World War.* Manchester University Press, 2012.

Leneman, Leah. *In the Service of Life: The Story of Elsie Inglis and the Scottish Women's Hospitals.* Mercat Press, Edinburgh, 1994.

MacDonald, Lyn. *The Roses of No Man's Land.* Michael Joseph, 1980.

McGreal, Stephen. *The War on Hospital Ships, 1914–1918.* Pen & Sword, Yorkshire, 2008.

Powell, Anne. *Women in the War Zone: Hospital Service in the First World War.* The History Press, Stroud, 2009.

Rees, Peter. *The Other ANZACS: Nurses at War, 1914–1918.* Allen & Unwin, 2008.

Riley-Smith, Jonathan. *Hospitallers: The History of The Order of St John.* Hambledon Press, 1999.

Scotland, Thomas and Heys, Steven (eds.). *War Surgery 1914–18.* Helion & Co, Solihull, 2012.

Wood, Emily. *The Red Cross Story.* Dorling Kindersley, 1995.

ARCHIVE COLLECTIONS

The National Archives, Kew, has more than 15,000 individual nursing service records available online. Website: www.nationalarchives.gov.uk/documentsonline/nursing.asp

The Imperial War Museum, London has an unparalleled collection of First World War material, including photographs, nurses and doctors diaries and correspondence, which can be viewed in the reading room. Wesbite: www.iwmcollections.org.uk

The Library of the Religious Society of Friends in Britain, Friends House, 173 Euston Road, London, NW1 2BJ, holds archive material and images relating to the Friends' Ambulance Unit in the First World War. Tel. 020 7663 1135. Website: www.quaker.org.uk/library

The Wellcome Archives, Wellcome Library, London, has a large collection of material related to medical services in the First World War, including field ambulance diaries, correspondence and official material. Website: www.wellcomelibrary.org

First World War material in *The Liddle Collection* in the Brotherton Library, University of Leeds, consists of around 5,000 collections of personal papers, including memoirs, photographs, diaries and interviews with medical personnel. There is an extensive online catalogue, and material can be viewed by appointment. Website: http://brs.leeds. ac.uk/~lib6osp/liddle.html

WEBSITES

The Long Long Trail has sections devoted to the medical treatment of casualties: www.1914-1918.net

Sue Light's website is an excellent source of information about British military nurses and all aspects of wartime nursing from 1880 onwards: www.scarletfinders.co.uk

David Cohen Fine Art specialises in art and ephemera of the First World War: www.davidcohenfineart.com

Lost Hospitals of London has a section devoted to the lost military hospitals of London: http://ezitis.myzen.co.uk

The website www.findmypast.co.uk has an area devoted to military nurses who served between approximately 1856 and 1994.

For a multimedia history of the First World War, view www.firstworldwar.com

The website of *Queen Alexandra's Royal Army Nursing Corps* has useful historical information about QAIMNS in the First World War: www.qaranc.co.uk

The Gillies Archive from Queen Mary's Hospital Sidcup is the most complete archive of medical notes from the First World War in the world: www. gilliesarchives.org.uk

For the *RAMC* in the First World War, with links to many other useful sites: www.ramc-ww1.com

The worldwide *Western Front Association* aims to perpetuate the memory, courage and comradeship of all those who fought on all sides and who served their countries during the Great War, including medical services: www.westernfrontassociation.com

GLOSSARY

ADS   Advanced Dressing Stations
BRC   British Red Cross
CCS   Casualty Clearing Station
FA   Field Ambulance
FANY   First Aid Nursing Yeomanry
FAU   Friends' Ambulance Unit
JWC   Joint War Committee
MSA   Millicent Sutherland Ambulance
OSJ   Order of St John
QAIMNS   Queen Alexandra's Imperial Military Nursing Service
RAMC   Royal Army Medical Corps
RAP   Regimental Aid Post
RMO   Regimental Medical Officer
TFNS   Territorial Force Nursing Service
VAD   Voluntary Aid Detachment
WHC   Women's Hospital Corps
WO   War Office

In 1916 the Manor House Estate was commandeered by the War Office and given to the Allied Hospital Benevolent Fund to build a hospital for injured servicemen. The hospital, in north-west London, opened in 1917 with 102 beds housed in temporary huts and its administration located in the Manor House. Note the standard-issue uniform.

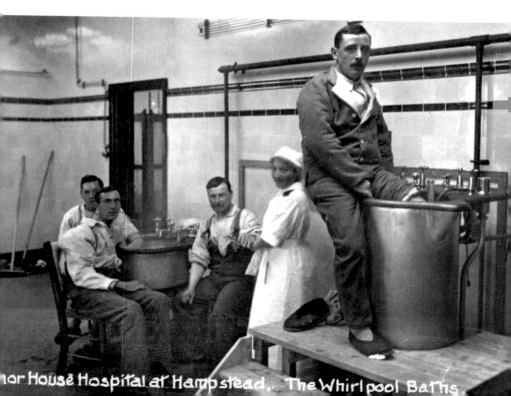

nor House Hospital at Hampstead. The Whirlpool Baths

INDEX

Page numbers in italics refer to illustrations

Aid posts: regimental 14, 27; first-aid
  28, *32*, 33, 35
Almeric Paget 55
Anaesthesia 21, 48
Awards 5, *8*, 33, 57–9, *58-9*
Battles: Mons 29, 39; Scarpe *29;*
  Somme 31; Ypres 31
Boer war 5
Brighton Pavilion *53*
Brittain, Vera 11
British Expeditionary Force (BEF) 19,
  37, 39, 41, 45, 57,
British Journal of Nursing 21, 24
British Red Cross Society (BRC) *3*, 5,
  8, 11, 16, *21*, *25*, 33, *34*, *35*, 39, 40,
  41, 48, 53, 57, *59*
Browne, Miss Sidney *7, 59*
Casualty clearing stations (CCS) 25,
  29, 30, 31, *31*, 36, 39
Casualties 15, 23, 27, *28,* 29, *29, 30*
  (top), 31, 40–1, 43, *44*, 45, 51
Chain of evacuation 26-31, 45
Chavasse, Noel Godfrey *56*, 57
Chisholm, Mairi 'Gipsy' 14, *32*, 33,
  35, 40, 58
Civil Hospital Reserve 5
Clark, Dr Hilda 17
Curie, Marie *24*
de Walden, Lady Howard 45
Doctors 15, 16, *16*, 17, 19, *19*, 21, *21*,
  23, 24, *26*, 27–8, 33, *40*, 41, *42*, 43,
  46-7, *56*, 57, *59*; women doctors 16,
  16, 17, 34–6, *37*, 58
Dressing stations 29
Eastern Front *12*
Field ambulance (FA) 20, 22, 27, 46, *47*
First Aid Nursing Yeomanry (FANY) 6,
  7, *10*, 11, 14, 20, 39, *40*, 58
First aid post *32*, 33, 35
French Flag Nursing Corps 14, 41, 59
Friends' Ambulance Unit (FAU) 15, *15*,
  38, 39, 58;
    Emergency and War Victims Relief
    Committee 17
Gallipoli 45-6, *46*
Garrett Anderson, Dr Louisa 16,
  24–5, 51
Gillies, Dr Harold 53
Haldane, Lord 5
Hospitals: Britain *3*, *8*, 11, 22, 43,

51–3, *52–3,* Eastern Front 45, 47–9;
  field 27; Western Front *10*, 11, 12–
  15, *15*, 17, 20, *21*, 24–5, *32*, 33, 34,
  34, *35*, *35*, 36–7 37, 51–5, *51–5*
Inglis, Dr Elsie *16*, 48
Ivens, Miss Frances 36, *37*, 58
Joint War Committee (JWC) 11, 15,
  16, 39, 48, 53
Keogh, Sir Alfred *4*, 5, 11, 17, 33, 35,
  39, 45, 51
Kitchener, Lord 19, 39
Knocker, Elsie 14, *32*, 33, 35, 40, 58
Martin-Leake, Arthur 57
Maude, Dr Dorothea Clara 17, 21, 48
McCarthy, Miss Maud 11, *13*, 36,
  57, *59*
McDougall, Grace, née Ashley-Smith 14
Medical conditions: amputation 19,
  24, 31, *50*, 51; blood transfusion
  25; chlorine gas 23–4; cholera *21;*
  consumption 52; diptheria 47;
  dysentery 52; fractures 23, *23;*
  frostbite 20, 35; gangrene 14, 19,
  25; lice 19, pneumonia; scarlet fever
  47; trench fever; trench foot 19, *20,*
  20; septicaemia 52; shell shock 21;
  typhoid *18,* 19, 47; typhoid (enteric)
  fever 19, *20,* 52; typhus 24; venereal
  disease 52
Millicent Sutherland Ambulance (MSA)
  13, *15*, 25
Mond, Captain Francis Leopold *2*
Munro, Dr Hector, Flying Ambulance
  Corps 13, 35, 40
Murray, Dr Flora 25, 51–2, *54*
Neilson-Gray, Norah *37*
Nurses/nursing 5-6, *6, 7, 8,* 11–14, *15*,
  16, 21, *22*, 27, 33, 37; individual
  nurses: Edith Appleton 31; Edith
  Cavell *12*; Sybil Cooke 24, Kate
  Finzi 12, 30-1; Evelyn Vickers Foote
  45; Katherine Furse 6, 13, 14; Miss
  Hastings 11, Elsie Knocker 14, *32*,
  33, 35, 40, 58; Miss Kate Luard
  12, 24, Joan Martin-Nicholson 12;
  Miss Maynard *14,* Mildred Rees 41;
  Miss Margaret Ripley 15, *31*; Flora
  Sandes 14; Mary Stevenson 43; Pat
  Waddell 20
Order of St John (OSJ) 5, 11
Paget, Lady 47-8
Queen Alexandra's Imperial Nursing

Service (QAIMNS) 5, 11, 13, *13,* 31,
  37, *42*, *59*; reserve 5, 6, 11, 41
Queen Victoria Jubilee Institute for
  Nurses 11, 43
Reckitt, Harold 36
Royal Army Medical Corps (RAMC)
  15, *16*, 17, 19, *20*, 21, *26*, 27
Sanitation 19, 48
Sassoon, Siegfried 53
*Scheme for the Organisation of Voluntary
  Aid* 5
Scottish Women's Hospital (SWH) *16*,
  17, 24, 36, *37*, 47–9, 58
Serbian Relief Fund 47–8
Sloggett, Sir Arthur Thomas 11, *12*, 39
Society of Friends *38*, 39, 58
Spencer, Stanley 52
St John Ambulance 33, 48, *58*
Stanley, Sir Arthur 15
Stobart, Mrs Mabel St. Clair 6, 33,
  47, 58
Stoney, Dr Florence 34
Stretchers: bearers 19, 27, *28*, 29, 46;
  cases *29*, 51
Territorial Force Nursing Service
  (TFNS) 5, 6, 7, 11, 59
Tonks, Henry *21*
Transport *43*: ambulance trains 37,
  38, 39, 41, *42*, 43, *43*; horse drawn
  ambulances 20, 30, 39, *40*, *46*;
  motor ambulances 15, 24, *29, 30,*
  39, 40, *40*, 41, 46, 58; hospital barge
  41, *42*; ships 41, 42, 43, *43*, *44*, 45
Trenches *9*, 14, 19, 20, *20*, 27, 29,
  35, 46
Vaccination *18*, 19, *20*
Voluntary Aid Detachments (VADs) 5,
  6, *8*, 11, 13, *14*, *16*, 33, 37, 39, 41,
  43, 45, 53, *55*, 57, *58*
War Office (WO) 5, 11, 14, 16, *17*, 33,
  35, 39, 55, *59*
Western Front *13*
Women's Emergency Corps 14
Women's Hospital Corps 16
Women's Sick and Wounded Convoy
  Corps 6, 9
Wounds 19–25, 27, 41, 47, *50*, 51,
  52, 53, 57
X-rays 24, *24*, 25, *25*, 31, 35, 47